Script Magic

A Hypnotherapist's Desk Reference

Clinical and Transpersonal Scripts
That Work Like Magic!

Second Revised Edition

Allen S. Chips, D.C.H., Ph.D.
and others

Coauthors/Contributors:
Masud Ansari, PhD, DCH
Marjorie Reynolds, PhD
Henry Leo Bolduc, CHt
Sydney Getchow, MHt
Kim Zapf, CHt
Rich Haas, CHt
Marc McGahee, MHt
Keith Clark, DCH
with permission from each of the authors/contributors
who currently maintain the rights to their scripts.

Editor:
Dee Chips

Original Cover Artwork by Allen S. Chips © 2001
Unattributed quotations are by Allen S. Chips

First Edition: August, 2001
First Revised Edition: January, 2003
Second Edition: August, 2004
Second Revised Edition: March, 2008

ISBN: 978-1-929661-06-0

Library of Congress Control Number: 2008923153

All Transpersonal Publishing titles are available at special quantity discounts directly from the publisher for sales promotions, mail order, conferences, and educational or institutional use. Special book excerpts or customized printings can also be created to fit specific needs. For details, contact the publisher:

Transpersonal Publishing
PO Box 7220
Kill Devil Hills, NC 27948
Orders: www.TranspersonalPublishing.com
(800) 296-MIND

Distributed by SCB distributors and available through all major wholesalers and bookstores

Printed in the United States of America

Script Magic
A Hypnotherapist's Desk Reference
(Second Revised Edition)

Dedication

In memory of Thomas Bacho
A great hypnotherapist and a dedicated assistant and friend
who transitioned in March 2004.

Thank You

To my editor and proof reader and those who have donated scripts to this book for the purpose of passing on the valuable benefits that hypnotherapy scripts provide.

Introduction

This book was put together as a tool for relaxation therapists, and primarily for clinical hypno-therapists. The most successful ways that hypnotherapists have been known to utilize hypnotherapy scripts are mentioned within the beginning pages of this book. In order to gain a greater understanding behind the use of these scripts, and thus becoming more effective with their use, the primary author of *Script Magic* recommends that the reader/therapist further research the causative factors behind the problems that are often helped with hypnotherapy. It is beneficial that individuals read or purchase additional texts, such as the ones that are listed on the "reference page" at the back of this book, in order to research the most beneficial hypnotherapeutic approaches for various interventions. Particularly in the case of hypnotic regression, it is very important readers educate themselves on various integrative models for the information that a client brings forward. To find an updated list of various texts on sug-gestive and regressive approaches that are available for purchase call 800-296-MIND, or log onto http://www.holistictree.com.

A "Flowchart for Hypnotherapy Sessions," which is followed by most hypnotherapists, is in-cluded in the beginning pages of this book. Both beginning and advanced suggestive therapists utilize a wide variety of suggestive therapy scripts in their private sessions, such as the ones contained within this book. However, most regression therapists also have other advanced methodologies that assist in creat-ing change, once a client is regressed into past memories. These advanced methodologies are taught at a variety of institutes throughout the United States. These institutes may be found through holistic directo-ries in one's local library, or by contacting the publisher. Often, the books that are listed on the reference page contain information on how to contact the author for various workshops and vocational opportuni-ties in the afterword pages.

Disclaimer

All of the authors of this book have given any person who wants to use these scripts permission to use them freely for private practice, or client sessions. This use includes "individual taping," which means that the scripts may be recorded exclusively for one individual at a time, and not mass-produced, or produced for resale. The authors give full permission to any person who desires to use these scripts for individual or group therapy. However, even though these scripts have been known by the authors to bring about positive results, the publisher and the authors have no control over the utilization and appli-cation of these. Who utilizes these scripts with whom, or how they are used is uncontrolled by the authors and publishers so these entities and persons are in no way responsible for the results of their use. It is advisable that each therapist and their client use discernment as to the utilization of the scripts listed within.

Future Editions

Occasionally, Script Magic will be revised with the addition of new scripts, building its pages year after year with more and more interventions that will create increased success for the clinical and transper-sonal hypnotherapist. Wholesale quantities of Script Magic may be acquired at TranspersonalPublishing.com. Retail copies of Script Magic may be acquired at http://www.holistictree.com. Readers may find Script Magic on CD-Rom to be very beneficial for adjusting the scripts and better serving the needs of themselves and their clients; the CD is available through the wholesale and retail web sites listed above.

Ways to Use Scripts

This section entails my opinions and practices derived from years of clinical research and private practice sessions that I've conducted. Some scripts were designed to be used back-to-back as two-session interventions, while others may be used as one-session interventions. The scripts utilized in sequence are listed as I and II, indicating the first and second session.

The weight loss scripts are put into two categories: general weight loss I and II; and several specialty scripts. The latter may be utilized in addition to I and II within a nine session (nine week) weight loss program for individual clients with weight reduction goals of approximately fifty pounds or greater. However, for goals less than this, it may be best to use the two general weight loss scripts once each week, within a two week program.

I have found most suggestive therapy sessions to be most successful when they revolve around two sessions—a week apart, particularly for smoking cessation. Session-one scripts are designed to create a completely new awareness and immediate life-style change. Session-two scripts are intended to instill the changes that have been accomplished from the first session. Frequently, session-two also contains suggestions to "tweak" anything that has not yet changed, relative to the therapeutic goal. In general, session-two is geared toward assisting the client with maintaining a confident attitude about the "permanent changes" that have taken place, as opposed to the attitude that only a "temporary change" has occurred (e.g. temporarily abstaining from cigarettes). This information was emphasized, because it may be necessary to create suggestions on the second session from scratch, in order to respond to the first session.

If a hypnotherapist does not have a good client interview method for extracting information from the client and thereby creating suggestions, it may be advisable to buy the book, *Clinical Hypnotherapy: A Transpersonal Approach*. It has an entire chapter on client interview methods for sessions one and two. The book proves to be a good complement to this writing and can be found on the publisher's page in the back of this book or through any major bookstore.

Creating suggestions on-the-fly will be necessary and is certainly able to be accomplished with a little creativity, of which every human being inherently has...the ability to create. This is how all of the scripts in this book have been developed, by hypnotherapists listening to various clients over many years and creating suggestions that have resulted in helping them, again and again. Enjoy the successes you'll obtain from this wonderful cooperative piece of therapeutic art known as *Script Magic*.

Session Flow Chart

Client Interview

↓

Hypnotic Induction

↓

Deepening Technique(s)

↓

Therapy: (Suggestive Script or Regression Script)

↓

Awakening Procedures

Deepening Techniques

Numbers Script- "OK now, when I count from one to ten, you will go one thousand times deeper, one hundred times deeper with each number you hear without even trying. One, and one hundred times deeper. Two, two hundred. Three...farther. Four...four hundred. Five...deeper. Six...(pause) Seven....and seven hundred. Eight...deeper. Nine...(pause) and Ten... one thousand times more deeply relaxed."

Scales/Yard Stick Script- "I want you to imagine a yardstick with your favorite color. Inch number thirty six represents your lightest state of relaxation and inch number one is the deepest. The next time I say the word "slide," I want you to go down toward the number one, your deepest level. Slide down now to the number one. Slide all the way down. Slide down, very deep."

Breathing Script- "...and now with each breath that you take, allow yourself to become more deeply relaxed...simply deeper with each breath...inhaling the light of relaxation and exhaling any tensions or tightness so that you may go deeper, (pause), deeper, (pause), and even deeper.

Finger Signal Script- "You know where your deepest level of relaxation is, so I will pause for a couple of minutes and you'll be able to go there automatically. You'll be able to raise your index finger when you get there. It may even flicker by itself to let you know you are at your deepest level...Go there now."

Pause Script- "I'm going to be silent for a couple of minutes. During that time, you can allow yourself to go much deeper into a state of deep relaxation, automatically, all on your own."

Steps Script- "Imagine that there's a safe flight of stairs before you... ten stairs... I'm going to count from one to ten, and when I reach the number ten, you'll be at your deepest level of relaxation. Take the first step at One. Two, deeper. Three... Four, farther. Five... Six... Seven... Eight... Nine... Ten. Deeply Relaxed."

Elevator Script- "Imagine that you are on the tenth floor of the building of relaxation. There's a safe elevator that can transport you to the basement level, which is the deepest level of relaxation. The elevator doors open and you step onto it, press the "B" button, for basement, and it starts gradually descending. Deeper...deeper... and deeper, all the way down to the basement level. The doors open and there's a hallway that leads you to go even deeper as you walk down the hallway..."

Escalator Script- "Imagine that there's an escalator before you. The escalator will take you to your deepest level of relaxation. As you step onto the escalator, it takes you there now (long pause). And you continue to go to deeper floors and deeper levels, then you get off at the deepest level."

Floating Script- "Imagine that you are floating toward your deepest level. Because you know where that deepest level is, you will simply feel yourself float there when I count from one to five. One, floating. Two, farther. Three, more relaxed. Four, deeper. And Five, deeply relaxed."

Fractionation Script- "I'm going to count back from three to one. When I reach the number one, you will briefly awaken, but when I snap my fingers like this (snap fingers), you will be able to close your eyes and go much deeper than before. Again...I'm going to count back from three to one. When I reach the number one, you will briefly awaken, but when I snap my fingers like this (snap fingers), you will be able to close your eyes and go much deeper than before. Three, more in touch with the room around you now. Two, the mind and body are returning back toward normal. And one, open your eyes, just briefly open your eyes now and (snap fingers). Deeper, deeper, and even deeper than before. Farther... Deeper with each breath...(pause)." [Repeat this three to five times from the beginning.]

Ambiguity Script- "What will happen from here is that my voice will get louder and then softer, and sometimes you won't be able to understand the words consciously, but your subconscious mind will absorb them any way. It will understand the words without even trying, automatically. Your conscious mind will sometimes hear the words, and sometimes it won't. So now you can go deeper with each breathe, automatically, you're going deeper and... so... it's... yes... and that's... because there's deep.... relaxa... (mumbling softly)... deep... slee... farth... (now become more loud) as you feel the body rest deeply, simply letting go, it falls loose and limp and the mind goes to that place of deep peace, farther, (mumbling softly), so that... and.. slee... relax... farther... and it even... yes... and that's how far... deeper.. (ramble words together).

Reframing The Conscious Mind Script- "Now the conscious mind needs to be acknowledged for its wonderful ability to rationalize, analyze, and make decisions about what's happening, but we're going to ask it to do these things later. We're asking it to wait until after the session to do these things, so that the subconscious mind can still receive suggestions in the form of images. It's going to move aside now, so that the subconscious is able to imagine things now. Even if it seems like it's making it up, the subconscious mind's job is to imagine in the form of pictures, sounds, and feelings. The conscious mind can simply move aside and do its thing, while the subconscious can do its job of simply just imagining things."

Double Bind Script- "You have a choice to either go to your deepest level right now, or you could wait just a few minutes until the end of this exercise to do so. Either way, you are going to go to your deepest level of relaxation. Remember what it feels like to be very, very deeply relaxed. Remember a time when the body was very tired at the end of the day and you laid down and let it just melt into the pads that you were laying against, as all the muscles relaxed at once, totally relaxing and content to be relaxing that deeply. And your mind just wanted to let go, completely. So you let it wander into a deep, distant direction, of deep, deep sleep (pause). Imagine that deep, deep, state of relaxation for the next few moments."

Rehearsal Script- "When I say the word "sleep," it simply means that you imagine what it would be like to become so relaxed that you experience a relaxation level that is as deep as the sleep state. Imagine what it would be like to be asleep. So sleep now. Sleep... Sleep... Deeper, asleep. Sleep... Sleep. Imagine a pleasant unconsciousness where there are no thoughts, now. A pleasant unconsciousness... Unconsciousness... deeper, into, unconsciousness... Unconsciousness... Sleep... Sleep."

Fear of Bridges

You have come to a point in your life where you are preparing to move beyond your fear of bridges. You are tired of feeling fear, so you are going to teach your mind and body to stop this unconscious reaction, to stop it and focus on relaxation instead. You will have an innate ability to relax in any situation from this day forward. The suggestion to relax will go deep into your unconscious mind, now. Relax... breathe deeply and easily, and now you will train your mind and body to experience relaxation while crossing a bridge. Train your mind to think of a very relaxing place, where you were very content and relaxed. You think now only about this place where you are happy. As you imagine this place, you can notice some colors there that are relaxing for you there in your surroundings. You can imagine some sounds that are relaxing for you to hear now. You can imagine a feeling of peace and relaxation in your body. The environment is just right, the temperature perfect. You are totally relaxed now, as you imagine your beautiful surroundings there. Notice how you can see, hear, or feel your safe-place there. You feel very natural there.

Now locate this very peaceful place in your body. This beautiful and natural place of peace is also stored in your body. Notice how you can locate this memory within your self and it makes you relax... relax naturally and automatically. Whenever you think of this safe-place, you relax automatically. Notice that you know where this memory is in your body and you are going to move this peaceful memory to the location in the body where you used to feel your fear. You move it to the place where you used to feel the fear. The fear feeling in the body disperses now. It is replaced with this very peaceful feeling, the peaceful memory. The peace grows within you. You have a right to feel peaceful. You have a right to be calm. Your body is now trained to respond to your ability to simply think about your safe-place. You think about it, you locate it in your body, and you're there. You feel relaxed. Whenever you think about your place of peace, you will relax. Regardless of where you are, you will relax automatically. Your mind will remember feelings of peace, relaxation, contentment, and you will relax anywhere at any time. You will unconsciously and automatically relax.

Now imagine that you are in the future. You are crossing a bridge, and you would have normally felt anxious but you feel relaxed. You think about your place of peace in your mind. You think about your place of peace in your body, and you are relaxed, as you cross the bridge. You are relaxed. You are relaxing in the future situation where you used to feel fear, but instead you are relaxed, content, at peace. You breathe deeply, but slowly. You know there is plenty of air, breathing easily & relaxed. You are relaxed and you feel great because you are crossing a bridge and feeling relaxed. Imagine how wonderful you feel as you cross the bridge. You feel self assured, confident, relaxed, and successful. You feel an exhilaration from succeeding at this with very little fear, or fear free, as you cross the bridge. Afterward, you have a wonderful feeling of success, self accomplishment, and a wonderful sense of freedom.

You feel great even now, because just thinking about it now, you know you are more relaxed in the present with the whole idea. You are at peace. Your fear has disappeared. You let it go. You are relaxed now. You are in control, relaxed, confident, at peace with the idea. You're at peace with this... peacefully, relaxed.

Fear of Crowds

You have come to a point in your life where you are preparing to move beyond your fear of crowds. You are tired of feeling fear, so you are going to teach your mind and body to stop this unconscious reaction, to stop it and focus on relaxation instead. You will have an innate ability to relax in any situation, from this day forward. The suggestion to relax will go deep into your unconscious mind now. Relax... breathe deeply and easily, and now you will train your mind and body to relax while being within crowds. Train your mind to think of a very relaxing place, where you were very content and relaxed. You think now only about this place where you are happy. As you imagine this place, you can notice some colors there that are relaxing for you there in your surroundings. You can imagine some sounds that are relaxing for you to hear now. You can imagine a feeling of peace and relaxation in your body. The environment is just right, the temperature perfect. You are totally relaxed now, as you imagine your beautiful surroundings there. Notice how you can see, hear, or feel your safe-place there. You feel very natural there.

Now locate this very peaceful place in your body. This beautiful and natural place of peace is also stored in your body. Notice how you can locate this memory within your self and it makes you relax... relax naturally and automatically. Whenever you think of this safe-place, you relax automatically. Notice that you know where this memory is in your body and you are going to move this peaceful memory to the location in the body where you used to feel your fear. You move it to the place where you used to feel the fear. The fear feeling in the body disperses now. It is replaced with this very peaceful feeling, the peaceful memory. The peace grows within you. You have a right to feel peaceful. You have a right to be calm. Your body is now trained to respond to your ability to simply think about your safe-place. You think about it, you locate it in your body, and you're there. You feel relaxed. Whenever you think about your place of peace, you will relax. Regardless of where you are, you will relax automatically. Your mind will remember feelings of peace, relaxation, contentment, and you will relax anywhere at any time. You will unconsciously and automatically relax.

Now imagine that you are in the future. You are within a crowd, and you would have normally felt anxious but you feel relaxed. You think about your place of peace in your mind. You think about your place of peace in your body, and you are relaxed, as you relax within the crowd. You are relaxed. You are relaxing in the future situation where you used to feel fear, but instead you are relaxed, content, at peace. You are relaxed and you feel great because you are accomplishing your goals of being in a crowd of people and feeling relaxed. You breathe deeply, one breathe at a time; you breathe slowly. You know there is plenty of air available to you, so you relax your breathing, slow, even, easy breathing... relaxed. Imagine how wonderful you feel as you walk or stand comfortably within a crowd. You feel self assured, confident, relaxed, and successful. You feel an exhilaration from succeeding at this with very little fear, or fear-free, as you relax within a crowd. Afterward, you have a wonderful feeling of success, self accomplishment, and a wonderful sense of freedom.

You feel great even now, because just thinking about it now, you know you are more relaxed in the present with the whole idea. You are at peace. Your fear has disappeared. You let it go. You are relaxed now. You are relaxed, confident, at peace with the idea. You're at peace with this... peacefully, relaxed.

Fear of the Dark

You have come to a point in your life where you are preparing to move beyond your fear of the dark. You are tired of feeling fear, so you are going to teach your mind and body to stop this unconscious reaction, to stop it and focus on relaxation instead. You will have an innate ability to relax in any situation from this day forward. The suggestion to relax will go deep into your unconscious mind now. Relax... breathe deeply and easily, and now you will train your mind and body to relax in the dark. Train your mind to think of a very relaxing place, where you were very content and relaxed. You think now only about this place where you are happy. As you imagine this place, you can notice some colors there that are relaxing for you there in your surroundings. You can imagine some sounds that are relaxing for you to hear now. You can imagine a feeling of peace and relaxation in your body. The environment is just right, the temperature perfect. You are totally relaxed now, as you imagine your beautiful surroundings there. Notice how you can see, hear, or feel your safe-place there. You feel very natural there.

Now locate this very peaceful place in your body. This beautiful and natural place of peace is also stored in your body. Notice how you can locate this memory within your self and it makes you relax... relax naturally and automatically. Whenever you think of this safe-place, you relax automatically. Notice that you know where this memory is in your body and you are going to move this peaceful memory to the location in the body where you used to feel your fear. You move it to the place where you used to feel the fear. The fear feeling in the body disperses now. It is replaced with this very peaceful feeling, the peaceful memory. The peace grows within you. You have a right to feel peaceful. You have a right to be calm. Your body is now trained to respond to your ability to simply think about your safe-place. You think about it, you locate it in your body, and you're there. You feel relaxed. Whenever you think about your place of peace, you will relax. Regardless of where you are, you will relax automatically. Your mind will remember feelings of peace, relaxation, contentment, and you will relax anywhere at any time. You will unconsciously and automatically relax.

Now imagine that you are in the future. You are in the dark, and you would have normally felt anxious but you feel relaxed. You think about your safe place in your mind. You think about your place of peace in your body, and you are relaxed, as you relax within the dark. You are relaxed. You are relaxing in the future situation where you used to feel fear, but instead you are relaxed, content, at peace. You are relaxed and you feel great because you are accomplishing your goals of being in the dark and feeling relaxed. You breathe deeply, one breathe at a time; you breathe slowly. You know there is plenty of air available to you, so you relax your breathing, slow, even, easy breathing... relaxed. Imagine how wonderful you feel as you simply relax in the dark. You feel self assured, confident, relaxed, and successful. You feel an exhilaration from succeeding at this with very little fear, or fear-free, as you relax in the dark. Afterward, you have a wonderful feeling of success, self accomplishment, and a wonderful sense of freedom.

You feel great even now, because just thinking about it now, you know you are more relaxed in the present with the whole idea. You are at peace. Your fear has disappeared. You let it go. You are relaxed now. You are relaxed, confident, at peace with the idea. You're at peace with this... peacefully, relaxed.

Fear of Driving

You have come to a point in your life where you are preparing to move beyond your fear of driving. You are tired of feeling fear, so you are going to teach your mind and body to stop this unconscious reaction, to stop it and focus on relaxation instead. You will have an innate ability to relax in any situation from this day forward. The suggestion to relax will go deep into your unconscious mind now. Relax... breathe deeply and easily, and now you will train your mind and body to relax and focus while driving. Train your mind to think of a very relaxing place, where you were very content and relaxed. You think now only about this place where you are happy. As you imagine this place, you can notice some colors there that are relaxing for you there in your surroundings. You can imagine some sounds that are relaxing for you to hear now. You can imagine a feeling of peace and relaxation in your body. The environment is just right, the temperature perfect. You are totally relaxed now, as you imagine your beautiful surroundings there. Notice how you can see, hear, or feel your safe-place there. You feel very natural there.

Now I want you to find this very peaceful place in your body. This beautiful and natural place of peace is also stored in your body. Notice how you can locate this memory within your self and it makes you relax... relax naturally and automatically. Whenever you think of this safe-place, you relax automatically. Notice that you know where this memory is in your body and you are going to move this peaceful memory to the location in the body where you used to feel your fear. You move it to the place where you used to feel the fear. The fear feeling in the body disperses now. It is replaced with this very peaceful feeling, the peaceful memory. The peace grows within you. You have a right to feel peaceful. You have a right to be calm. Your body is now trained to respond to your ability to simply think about your safe-place. You think about it, you locate it in your body, and you're there. You feel relaxed. Whenever you think about your place of peace, you will relax. Regardless of where you are, you will relax automatically. Your mind will remember feelings of peace, relaxation, contentment, and you will relax anywhere at any time. You will unconsciously and automatically relax.

Now imagine that you are in the future. You are driving, and you would have normally felt anxious but you feel relaxed. You think about your safe place in your mind. You think about your place of peace in your body, and you are relaxed, as you relax and concentrate while driving. You are relaxed. You are relaxing in the future situation where you used to feel fear, but instead you are relaxed, content, at peace, with a higher level of concentration. You are relaxed and you feel great because you are accomplishing your goals of driving and feeling relaxed. You breathe deeply, one breath at a time; you breathe slowly. You know there is plenty of air available to you, so you relax your breathing, slow, even, easy breathing... relaxed. Imagine how wonderful you feel as you simply relax while driving and you're aware of everything around you, having a focused concentration level. You feel safe. You feel self assured, confident, relaxed, and successful. You feel an exhilaration from succeeding at this with very little fear, or fear-free, as you relax while driving. Afterward, you have a wonderful feeling of success, self accomplishment, and a wonderful sense of freedom.

You feel great even now, because just thinking about it now, you know you are more relaxed in the present with the whole idea. You are at peace. Your fear has disappeared. You let it go. You are relaxed now. You are relaxed, confident, at peace with the idea. You're at peace with this... peacefully, relaxed.

Fear of Enclosed Spaces

You have come to a point in your life where you are preparing to move beyond your fear of enclosed spaces. You are tired of feeling fear, so you are going to teach your mind and body to stop this unconscious reaction, to stop it and focus on succeeding and being relaxed instead. You will have an innate ability to relax in any situation from this day forward. The suggestion to relax will go deep into your unconscious mind now. Relax... breathe deeply and easily, and now you will train your mind and body to relax and focus while being in enclosed spaces. Train your mind to think of a very relaxing place, where you were very content and relaxed. You think now only about this place where you are happy. As you imagine this place, you can notice some colors there that are relaxing for you there in your surroundings. You can imagine some sounds that are relaxing for you to hear now. You can imagine a feeling of peace and relaxation in your body. The environment is just right, the temperature perfect. You are totally relaxed now, as you imagine your beautiful surroundings there. Notice how you can see, hear, or feel your safe-place there. You feel very natural there.

Now I want you to find this very peaceful place in your body. This beautiful and natural place of peace is also stored in your body. Notice how you can locate this memory within your self and it makes you relax... relax naturally and automatically. Whenever you think of this safe-place, you relax automatically. Notice that you know where this memory is in your body and you are going to move this peaceful memory to the location in the body where you used to feel your fear. You move it to the place where you used to feel the fear. The fear feeling in the body disperses now. It is replaced with this very peaceful feeling, the peaceful memory. The peace grows within you. You have a right to feel peaceful. You have a right to be calm. Your body is now trained to respond to your ability to simply think about your safe-place. You think about it, you locate it in your body, and you're there. You feel relaxed. Whenever you think about your place of peace, you will relax. Regardless of where you are, you will relax automatically. Your mind will remember feelings of peace, relaxation, contentment, and you will relax anywhere at any time. You will unconsciously and automatically relax.

Now imagine that you are in the future. You are within an enclosed space, and you would have normally felt anxious but you feel relaxed. You think about your safe place in your mind. You think about your place of peace in your body, and you are relaxed, as you relax and concentrate while being in an enclosed space. You are relaxed. You are relaxing in the future situation where you used to feel fear, but instead you are relaxed, content, at peace, with a higher level of concentration. You are relaxed and you feel great because you are accomplishing your goals of being in an enclosed space and feeling relaxed. You breathe deeply, one breath at a time; you breathe slowly. You know there is plenty of air available to you, so you relax your breathing, slow, even, easy breathing... relaxed. Imagine how wonderful you feel as you simply relax while within an enclosed space and you're aware of everything around you, having a focused concentration level. You feel safe. You feel self assured, confident, relaxed, and successful. You feel an exhilaration from succeeding at this with very little fear, or fear-free, as you relax within enclosed spaces. Afterward, you have a wonderful feeling of success, self accomplishment, and a wonderful sense of freedom.

You feel great even now, because just thinking about it now, you know you are more relaxed in the present with the whole idea. You are at peace. Your fear has disappeared. You let it go. You are relaxed now. You are relaxed, confident, at peace with the idea. You're at peace with this... peacefully, relaxed.

Fear of Failure

You have come to a point in your life where you are preparing to move beyond your fear of failure. You are tired of not even giving yourself a chance to succeed, so you are going to teach your mind and body to stop this unconscious reaction, to stop it and focus on trying something new and what it would be like to succeed. The suggestion to "relax and give it a try" will go deep into your unconscious mind now. Relax... breathe deeply and easily, and now you will train your mind and body to relax and focus on the ability to try new things. Train your mind to think of a time when you've succeeded at something in the past, where you tried something new and it worked out perfectly. You think now only about this memory where you are happy and thankful to yourself for trying and succeeding. As you imagine this time, you can notice some colors there that represent this. You can imagine some sounds that are relaxing for you there. You can imagine a feeling of peace and relaxation in your body. The environment is just right there. You are totally relaxed now, as you imagine your successful surroundings there. Notice how you can see, hear, or feel your success there. You feel very natural there.

Now locate this feeling of success in your body. You can locate this memory within your self and it makes you relax... relax naturally and automatically. Whenever you think of it, you relax automatically. Notice that you know where this memory is in your body and you are going to move this successful memory to the location in the body where you used to feel fear. You move it to the place where you used to feel the fear. The fear feeling in the body disperses now. It is replaced with this very peaceful feeling, the peaceful memory. The peace grows within you. You have a right to try to accomplish things just as much as anybody else. You have a right to try to be successful at anything. You think about it, you locate it in your body, and you're there. You feel relaxed. Whenever you think about your success memory, you will relax. Regardless of where you are, you will relax automatically. Your mind will remember feelings of peace, relaxation, contentment, and you will know that you can be successful anywhere at any time. You will unconsciously and automatically relax and focus with being successful.

Now imagine that you are in the future. You are experiencing a time when you would have normally felt anxious about it, but instead you feel relaxed. You think about your past success in your mind. You concentrate on your natural abilities, your creative resources, while knowing you are capable of being successful. You are relaxed with the idea. You are relaxing in the future situation where you used to feel fear, but instead you are relaxed, content, at peace, with a higher level of concentration. You are relaxed and you feel great because you are accomplishing your goals, as you know all concerns will disappear quickly and naturally. You breathe deeply, one breath at a time; you breathe slowly. You know there is plenty of air available to you, so you relax your breathing, slow, even, easy breathing... relaxed. Imagine how wonderful you feel as you simply relax with the idea that you have the ability to be successful, having a focused concentration level. You feel safe. You feel self assured, confident, relaxed, and successful. You know that everything is going to be OK this time. You feel an exhilaration from succeeding at this with little concern, or practically fear-free, as you relax and let all concerns pass. Afterward, you have a wonderful feeling of success, self accomplishment, and a wonderful sense of freedom.

You feel great even now, because just thinking about it now, you know you are more relaxed with the whole idea. You are at peace and in control. Your fear has disappeared. You let it go. You are relaxed now. You are relaxed, confident, at peace with the idea. You're at peace with this... peacefully, relaxed.

Fear of Fear Itself

You have come to a point in your life where you are preparing to move beyond your fear of experiencing fear. You are tired of feeling fear, so you are going to teach your mind and body to stop this unconscious reaction, to stop it and focus on succeeding and being relaxed instead. You will have an innate ability to relax in any situation from this day forward. The suggestion to relax will go deep into your unconscious mind now. Relax... breathe deeply and easily, and now you will train your mind and body to relax and focus while allowing yourself to feel a little fear and relax with it. Train your mind to think of a very relaxing place, where you were very content and relaxed. You think now only about this place where you are happy. As you imagine this place, you can notice some colors there that are relaxing for you there in your surroundings. You can imagine some sounds that are relaxing for you to hear now. You can imagine a feeling of peace and relaxation in your body. The environment is just right, the temperature perfect. You are totally relaxed now, as you imagine your beautiful surroundings there. Notice how you can see, hear, or feel your safe-place there. You feel very natural there.

Now I want you to find this very peaceful place in your body. This beautiful and natural place of peace is within you; you can locate this memory within your self and it makes you relax... relax naturally and automatically. Whenever you think of this safe-place, you relax automatically. Notice that you know where this memory is in your body and you are going to move this peaceful memory to the location in the body where you used to feel your fear. You move it to the place where you used to feel the fear. The fear feeling in the body disperses now. It is replaced with this very peaceful feeling, the peaceful memory. The peace grows within you. You have a right to feel peaceful. You have a right to be calm. Your body is now trained to respond to your ability to simply think about your safe-place. You think about it, you locate it in your body, and you're there. You feel relaxed. Whenever you think about your place of peace, you will relax. Regardless of where you are, you will relax automatically. Your mind will remember feelings of peace, relaxation, contentment, and you will relax anywhere at any time. You will unconsciously and automatically relax.

Now imagine that you are in the future. You are feeling the natural feeling of a little fear, and you would have normally felt anxious about it, but instead you feel relaxed. You think about your safe place in your mind. You think about your place of peace in your body, and you are relaxed, as you relax and concentrate while tolerating the natural feeling of fear. You are relaxed. You are relaxing in the future situation where you used to feel fear, but instead you are relaxed, content, at peace, with a higher level of concentration. You are relaxed and you feel great because you are accomplishing your goals of feeling a little bit of fear and feeling relaxed, because you know it will pass, it will pass. You breathe deeply, one breath at a time; you breathe slowly. You know there is plenty of air available to you, so you relax your breathing, slow, even, easy breathing... relaxed. Imagine how wonderful you feel as you simply relax and let natural feelings of fear simply pass, having a focused concentration level. You feel safe. You feel self assured, confident, relaxed, and successful. You feel an exhilaration from succeeding at this with very little fear, or fear-free, as you relax with the fear and let it pass. Afterward, you have a wonderful feeling of success, self accomplishment, and a wonderful sense of freedom.

You feel great even now, because just thinking about it now, you know you are more relaxed in the present with the whole idea. You are at peace and in control. Your fear has disappeared. You let it go. You are relaxed now. You are relaxed, confident, at peace with the idea. You're at peace with this... peacefully, relaxed.

Fear of Flying

You have come to a point in your life where you are preparing to move beyond your fear of flying. You are tired of feeling fear, so you are going to teach your mind and body to stop this unconscious reaction, to stop it and focus on succeeding and being relaxed instead. You will have an innate ability to relax in any situation from this day forward. The suggestion to relax will go deep into your unconscious mind now. Relax... breathe deeply and easily, and now you will train your mind and body to relax and focus while flying. Train your mind to think of a very relaxing place, where you were very content and relaxed. You think now only about this place where you are happy. As you imagine this place, you can notice some colors there that are relaxing for you there in your surroundings. You can imagine some sounds that are relaxing for you to hear now. You can imagine a feeling of peace and relaxation in your body. The environment is just right, the temperature perfect. You are totally relaxed now, as you imagine your beautiful surroundings there. Notice how you can see, hear, or feel your safe-place there. You feel very natural there.

Now locate this very peaceful place in your body. This beautiful and natural place of peace is within you; you can locate this memory within your self and it makes you relax... relax naturally and automatically. Whenever you think of this safe-place, you relax automatically. Notice that you know where this memory is in your body and you are going to move this peaceful memory to the location in the body where you used to feel your fear. You move it to the place where you used to feel the fear. The fear feeling in the body disperses now. It is replaced with this very peaceful feeling, the peaceful memory. The peace grows within you. You have a right to feel peaceful. You have a right to be calm. Your body is now trained to respond to your ability to simply think about your safe-place. You think about it, you locate it in your body, and you're there. You feel relaxed. Whenever you think about your place of peace, you will relax. Regardless of where you are, you will relax automatically. Your mind will remember feelings of peace, relaxation, contentment, and you will relax anywhere at any time. You will unconsciously and automatically relax.

Now imagine that you are in the future. You are boarding a plane and you would have normally felt anxious about it, but instead you feel relaxed. You think about your safe place in your mind. You think about your place of peace in your body, and you are relaxed. You relax and concentrate while focusing on relaxing ideas. You are relaxed. You are relaxing in the future situation where you used to feel fear, but instead you are relaxed, content, at peace, with a higher level of concentration. You are relaxed and you feel great because you are accomplishing your goals of flying and feeling relaxed, as you know all concerns will disappear quickly and naturally. You breathe deeply, one breath at a time; you breathe slowly. You know there is plenty of air available to you, so you relax your breathing, slow, even, easy breathing... relaxed. Imagine how wonderful you feel as you simply relax and start flying, having a focused concentration level. You feel safe. You feel self assured, confident, relaxed, and successful. You know that everything is going to be OK this time. You feel an exhilaration from succeeding at this with little concern, or practically fear-free, as you relax and let them pass. Afterward, you have a wonderful feeling of success, self accomplishment, and a wonderful sense of freedom.

You feel great even now, because just thinking about it now, you know you are more relaxed in the present with the whole idea. You are at peace and in control. Your fear has disappeared. You let it go. You are relaxed now. You are relaxed, confident, at peace with the idea. You're at peace with this... peacefully, relaxed.

17

Fear of Heights

You have come to a point in your life where you are preparing to move beyond your fear of heights. You are tired of feeling fear, so you are going to teach your mind and body to stop this unconscious reaction, to stop it and focus on succeeding and being relaxed instead. You will have an innate ability to relax in any situation from this day forward. The suggestion to relax will go deep into your unconscious mind now. Relax... breathe deeply and easily, and now you will train your mind and body to relax and focus around heights. Train your mind to think of a very relaxing place, where you were very content and relaxed. You think now only about this place where you are happy. As you imagine this place, you can notice some colors there that are relaxing for you there in your surroundings. You can imagine some sounds that are relaxing for you to hear now. You can imagine a feeling of peace and relaxation in your body. The environment is just right, the temperature perfect. You are totally relaxed now, as you imagine your beautiful surroundings there. Notice how you can see, hear, or feel your safe-place there. You feel very natural there.

Now locate this very peaceful place in your body. This beautiful and natural place of peace is within you; you can locate this memory within your self and it makes you relax... relax naturally and automatically. Whenever you think of this safe-place, you relax automatically. Notice that you know where this memory is in your body and you are going to move this peaceful memory to the location in the body where you used to feel your fear. You move it to the place where you used to feel the fear. The fear feeling in the body disperses now. It is replaced with this very peaceful feeling, the peaceful memory. The peace grows within you. You have a right to feel peaceful. You have a right to be calm. Your body is now trained to respond to your ability to simply think about your safe-place. You think about it, you locate it in your body, and you're there. You feel relaxed. Whenever you think about your place of peace, you will relax. Regardless of where you are, you will relax automatically. Your mind will remember feelings of peace, relaxation, contentment, and you will relax anywhere at any time. You will unconsciously and automatically relax.

Now imagine that you are in the future. You are experiencing a height and you would have normally felt anxious about it, but instead you feel relaxed. You think about your safe place in your mind. You think about your place of peace in your body, and you are relaxed, as you relax and concentrate while focusing on relaxing ideas. You are relaxed. You are relaxing in the future situation where you used to feel fear, but instead you are relaxed, content, at peace, with a higher level of concentration. You are relaxed and you feel great because you are accomplishing your goals of being up high and feeling relaxed, as you know all concerns will disappear quickly and naturally. You breathe deeply, one breath at a time; you breathe slowly. You know there is plenty of air available to you, so you relax your breathing, slow, even, easy breathing... relaxed. Imagine how wonderful you feel as you simply relax with heights, having a focused concentration level. You feel safe. You feel self assured, confident, relaxed, and successful. You know that everything is going to be OK this time. You feel an exhilaration from succeeding at this with little concern, or practically fear-free, as you relax and let all concerns pass. Afterward, you have a wonderful feeling of success, self accomplishment, and a wonderful sense of freedom.

You feel great even now, because just thinking about it now, you know you are more relaxed in the present with the whole idea. You are at peace and in control. Your fear has disappeared. You let it go. You are relaxed now. You are relaxed, confident, at peace with the idea. You're at peace with this... peacefully, relaxed.

Fear of Incontinence

You have come to a point in your life where you are preparing to move beyond your fear of incontinence. You are tired of feeling fear, so you are going to teach your mind and body to stop this unconscious reaction, to stop it and focus on recognizing when it's time to go and being relaxed about it instead. You will have an innate ability to hold yourself in any situation from this day forward. The suggestion to hold it will go deep into your unconscious mind now. Relax... breathe deeply and easily, and now you will train your mind and body to relax and focus on being able to get the signal early and hold off, hold off. Train your mind to think of a time when you could hold it successfully, where you were very confident that the body would work with you on this. You think now only about this time; you were happy about the body's ability to signal and hold-off. As you imagine this time, you can notice some colors there that are relaxing for you there in your surroundings. You can imagine some sounds that are relaxing for you to hear now. You can imagine a feeling of confidence within your body. The environment is just right, the temperature perfect. You are totally confident in the body's ability, as you imagine your surroundings there. Notice how you can see, hear, or feel that you are safe there. You feel very natural there.

Now imagine that you are in the future. You are experiencing a signal from the body and you would have normally felt anxious about it, but instead you feel relaxed because you can hold off, hold off, like turning a faucet off tight. You remember that you had this ability by holding tight after the signal, all the way off, turned off. You think about your ability, as you concentrate on how you will be able to relax and hold on. You are relaxing in the future situation where you used to feel fear, but instead you are relaxed, content, and confident, with a greater ability to shut it down. You are relaxed and you feel great because you are accomplishing your goals of holding off, longer and longer. You breathe deeply, one breath at a time; you breathe slowly. You know there is plenty of time to make it, so you relax your breathing, slow, even, easy breathing... relaxed. You know that everything is going to be OK this time. You only think of release when you get to the point where it's OK to do so. You put release out of your mind, you forget about it, until it's OK to do so. When it's OK, you will say "release" and at the right time, you will release. You feel an exhilaration from succeeding at this with little concern, or practically fear-free, as you relax and let all concerns pass. Afterward, you have a wonderful feeling of success, self accomplishment, and a wonderful sense of freedom.

You feel great even now, because just thinking about it now, you know you are more relaxed with the whole idea. You are at peace and in control. Your fear has disappeared. You let it go. You are relaxed now. You are relaxed, confident, at peace with the idea. You're at peace with this... peacefully, relaxed.

Fear of Water

You have come to a point in your life where you are preparing to move beyond your fear of water. You are tired of feeling fear, so you are going to teach your mind and body to stop this unconscious reaction...to stop it, and focus on feel normal. You will have an innate ability to relax yourself in any situation from this day forward. The suggestion to relax will go deep into your unconscious mind now. Relax... breathe deeply and easily, and now you will train your mind and body to relax and focus around water. Train your mind to think of a very relaxing place, where you were very content and relaxed. You think now only about this place where you are happy. As you imagine this place, you can notice some colors there that are relaxing for you there in your surroundings. You can imagine some sounds that are relaxing for you to hear now. You can imagine a feeling of peace and relaxation in your body. The environment is just right, the temperature perfect. You are totally relaxed now, as you imagine your beautiful surroundings there. Notice how you can see, hear, or feel your safe-place there. You feel very natural there.

Now locate this very peaceful place in your body. This beautiful and natural place of peace is within you; you can locate this memory within your self and it makes you relax... relax naturally and automatically. Whenever you think of this safe-place, you relax automatically. Notice that you know where this memory is in your body and you are going to move this peaceful memory to the location in the body where you used to feel your fear. You move it to the place where you used to feel the fear. The fear feeling in the body disperses now. It is replaced with this very peaceful feeling, the peaceful memory. The peace grows within you. You have a right to feel peaceful. You have a right to be calm. Your body is now trained to respond to your ability to simply think about your safe-place. You think about it, you locate it in your body, and you're there. You feel relaxed. Whenever you think about your place of peace, you will relax. Regardless of where you are, you will relax automatically. Your mind will remember feelings of peace, relaxation, contentment, and you will relax anywhere at any time. You will unconsciously and automatically relax.

Now imagine that you are in the future. You are exposed to water and you would have normally felt anxious about it, but instead you feel relaxed. You think about your safe place in your mind. You think about your place of peace in your body, and you are relaxed, as you relax and concentrate while focusing on relaxing ideas. You are relaxed. You are relaxing in the future situation where you used to feel fear, but instead you are relaxed, content, at peace, with a higher level of concentration. You are relaxed and you feel great because you are accomplishing your goals of being exposed to water and feeling relaxed, as you know all concerns will disappear quickly and naturally. You breathe deeply, one breath at a time; you breathe slowly. You know there is plenty of air available to you, so you relax your breathing, slow, even, easy breathing... relaxed. Imagine how wonderful you feel as you simply relax with the water, having a focused concentration level. You feel safe. You feel self assured, confident, relaxed, and successful. You know that everything is going to be OK this time. You feel an exhilaration from succeeding at this with little concern, or practically fear-free, as you relax and let all concerns pass. Afterward, you have a wonderful feeling of success, self accomplishment, and a wonderful sense of freedom.

You feel great even now, because just thinking about it now, you know you are more relaxed in the present with the whole idea. You are at peace and in control. Your fear has disappeared. You let it go. You are relaxed now. You are relaxed, confident, at peace with the idea. You're at peace with this... peacefully, relaxed.

Miscellaneous Fears

You have come to a point in your life where you are preparing to move beyond your fear of _____. You are tired of feeling fear, so you are going to teach your mind and body to stop this unconscious reaction. To stop it, and focus on feeling normal, composed, and succeeding and being relaxed. You will have an innate ability to relax in any situation from this day forward. The suggestion to relax will go deep into your unconscious mind now. Relax... breathe deeply and easily, and now you will train your mind and body to relax and focus around _____. Train your mind to think of a very relaxing place, where you were very content and relaxed. You think now only about this place where you are happy. As you imagine this place, you can notice some colors there that are relaxing for you there in your surroundings. You can imagine some sounds that are relaxing for you to hear now. You can imagine a feeling of peace and relaxation in your body. The environment is just right, the temperature perfect. You are totally relaxed now, as you imagine your beautiful surroundings there. Notice how you can see, hear, or feel your safe-place there. You feel very natural there.

Now locate this very peaceful place in your body. This beautiful and natural place of peace is within you; you can locate this memory within your self and it makes you relax... relax naturally and automatically. Whenever you think of this safe-place, you relax automatically. Notice that you know where this memory is in your body and you are going to move this peaceful memory to the location in the body where you used to feel your fear. You move it to the place where you used to feel the fear. The fear feeling in the body disperses now. It is replaced with this very peaceful feeling, the peaceful memory. The peace grows within you. You have a right to feel peaceful. You have a right to be calm. Your body is now trained to respond to your ability to simply think about your safe-place. You think about it, you locate it in your body, and you're there. You feel relaxed. Whenever you think about your place of peace, you will relax. Regardless of where you are, you will relax automatically. Your mind will remember feelings of peace, relaxation, contentment, and you will relax anywhere at any time. You will unconsciously and automatically relax.

Now imagine that you are in the future. You are experiencing a _____ and you would have normally felt anxious about it, but instead you feel relaxed. You think about your safe place in your mind. You think about your place of peace in your body, and you are relaxed, as you relax and concentrate while focusing on relaxing ideas. You are relaxed. You are relaxing in the future situation where you used to feel fear, but instead you are relaxed, content, at peace, with a higher level of concentration. You are relaxed, and you feel great because you are accomplishing your goals of _____ (future goal) and feeling relaxed, as you know all concerns will disappear quickly and naturally. You breathe deeply, one breath at a time; you breathe slowly. You know there is plenty of air available to you, so you relax your breathing, slow, even, easy breathing... relaxed. Imagine how wonderful you feel as you simply relax with the idea of _____ , having a focused concentration level. You feel safe. You feel self assured, confident, relaxed, and successful. You know that everything is going to be OK this time. You feel an exhilaration from succeeding at this with little concern, or practically fear-free, as you relax and let all concerns pass. Afterward, you have a wonderful feeling of success, self accomplishment, and a wonderful sense of freedom.

You feel great even now, because just thinking about it now, you know you are more relaxed in the present with the whole idea. You are at peace and in control. Your fear has disappeared. You let it go. You are relaxed now. You are relaxed, confident, at peace with the idea. You're at peace with this... peacefully, relaxed.

WEIGHT LOSS I

Remember that you're the one who put your foot down to make this change, so you'll take most of the credit. I'm like a guide an a backpacking trip showing you the way; you're still carrying your own backpack with important weight reduction goals that you know how to reach. So, when you're thin and you look back, you'll say to yourself, "I lost the weight"...And remember that this has *nothing to do with dieting;* we're simply creating new eating habits that are more satisfying for you each and every day. Never again will you deprive yourself of any food, such as in dieting; if you want it, within moderation, you can have it... a little bit here or a little bit there and you are completely satisfied. Yet, you'll find your desire for healthier food is enhanced.

By putting new eating habit suggestions into your subconscious mind, your subconscious urges will involve your desire to be thin. You are going to have the attitudes that thinner people have about eating. You're simply losing your appetite for fattening foods and overeating, yet you still feel like you're getting what you want with healthier foods; you're still getting what you need, with less food; you eat a reasonable portion of food and you are satisfied. This is the mind and body of a thinner person, and you are going to have the willpower to make healthy, thinner, happier decisions. You'll make healthier choices for yourself at the grocery store, restaurants, and at home. You will be aware of the right choices toward thinness everywhere you go. You are going to experience a sense of control over your own behavior now, with a greater will-power. You are going to be in control, stronger, self empowered to do the right thing for yourself. You are more confident now....more confident than ever before that you can do this thing. You are using the power of the subconscious mind to make the change and keep the change; the words, "I can do it this time" may even enter into your mind from time to time. You've seen others do it, and now you are ready to experience a fit and trim life-style.

As you create new eating habits that are more satisfying, you are going to become more realistic about your body's food consumption...

Food is simply a biochemical substance that sustains life in a biochemical machine called the body. Food outside of the body completely changes its appearance and texture; after it enters the mouth, the bones there, we call teeth, chop it up with secretions of saliva. Then it becomes a pasty substance that's flushed down and washed around in a bowl of acid we call the stomach. From there it becomes a milky substance that's absorbed into the intestinal walls and deposited into the designated areas of the body. As you become a more practical eater, you're losing your interest in meat. Most meats are about 70% fat, and the truth is, meat is nothing more than dead-animal muscle, so it's easy to avoid or reduce it. You'll reach an awareness therefore that food almost has a spiritual value to you now; as taste and eating is simply a process that was designed on a higher level in order to sustain life in a physical vehicle, the body, the temple for the spirit.

Remember that taste buds on the tongue were simply designed on a higher level to send perceptual signals to the brain. Enjoying your food was intended to sustain life in the body, but only in moderation. Your mind is the builder and the body is the result, so now your mind is building new realizations that will help you reduce your weight, such as that everybody has different past experiences that have programmed the sensory units on the tongue we call taste buds, which have created both healthy and problematic preferences for food. But these are only programmed perceptions. Now, you are going to de-program your past unhealthy habits of overeating, or eating too much fattening food. You're going to retrain your taste buds now to enjoy health, low-fat foods; fruits, vegetables, grains, and _____ and other thin alternatives. As you begin to sample many healthy foods, you notice you enjoy healthier foods more. You experiment with them, and over time, you are creative with seasonings and other healthy ways to make them taste better and you learn to like them. You're reducing your desire for processed sugar and flour, because flower and water make glue, and eating glue is unhealthy. Processed sugar in large quantities in unhealthy, so you notice you begin to lose your appetite for sugar and sugary foods. They simply taste too sweet. Notice how you reduce and then eliminate carbonated beverages and begin to train your taste buds to enjoy less and less sugary tasting drinks. Sugary drinks start to taste too sweet then, too sweet and you cut back.

And because everybody trains their taste buds in childhood, the things you were deprived of then are available to you all the time now. They mean nothing, because you have more than you need practically everywhere. All the stores, restaurants, even at home; they're all *stuffed full* of food, so it's easy to feel you have more than you want of any foods you were deprived of, or any "special" food from childhood. You have them all around you, and you could have them anytime you want, so it's no big deal just to skip them. Never again will anybody tell you what you can and can't have; that's just kid's stuff, so these foods lose their value. You can make the choice now; so if you've been told to clean your plate; the heck with that now. Nobody benefited from your overeating in the past, so you can waste it or save it for later. You can leave food on your plate without any guilt now.

You'll take smaller more reasonable portions now, knowing that if you were hungry after a small portion you could take another small one, but to your own amazement you've had enough. But if you should ever take too much, you are able to leave food on your plate now. You can let it go...you know your body doesn't need it. You are releasing your body from the shackles of overeating, pushing food away, or pushing away from the table or counter tops. And remember, you don't care what anybody else thinks, this is something you're *doing for yourself.* (list client's motivations)

As you're creating the habits of a thinner person, you're separating all feelings from problematic foods. You are taking back control by imagining attachments in the form of invisible energy cords to each problematic food.... and now you're cutting the cords, one at a time, reducing or eliminating the emotions behind them. The truth is, problematic foods have nothing to do with the way you feel anymore. Food has nothing to do with stresses, rewards, moods, loneliness, happiness, or any ups and downs through the natural course of living life. Now you've separated food from feelings, and there's a wonderful feeling of freedom.

Even at social occasions, you can turn down food without feeling rude or impolite. But notice how you still enjoy being sociable, enjoying your time with friends and family, just as you always have, but with smaller portions, healthier choices, and without overeating. This is a very personal choice, so you'll avoid letting anybody influence your new healthier eating habits. You'll ignore any friend's or family member's comments about your eating less or more healthy food in the beginning, unless they are supportive comments. You hear only supportive comments. Over time everybody with your best interest at heart will adjust to the new you. People will be impressed with the changes you've made in yourself; making positive comments about your looking good... and they'll respect you and your decisions more...Your attractive new image will serve as a positive role model for others, at work, home and when you go out places. You simply carry yourself differently, with a higher self image.

In the days ahead, you are going to start losing your appetite for heavier, fattening foods. You're going to imagine things you don't like about them. Fattening foods just don't sit right on the stomach as they seem to just sit there like a ball of glue; so you prefer lighter more quickly digestible foods. Sometimes, you'll notice things you dislike about fats—such as the overly-stuffed feeling, and the oily sensation on the tongue and throat. Fattening oils have the same consistency and texture as motor oil; so if you occasionally choose a fattening food, notice how you're able to eat small portions and you've had enough, you're completely satisfied. Small portions of sweets are enough for you, as you're reminded to reduce them with that sicky sweet taste in the back of the mouth from a time when you've eaten too many sweets. Your body is working with you now, telling you when to stop eating, and you're listening. You only eat when you are truly, physically hungry, which is only a couple of times a day. So you're promising to yourself now, "I will only eat when I'm truly hungry."

Remember that quality is more important than quantity, so it's logical to eat slower... very slowly... at meal times, chewing slowly and eating less food; people only taste 10% of the food that slides down the throat anyway—the rest is just stuffing, so you may find it more enjoyable to slowly savor small amounts of your favorite foods once in a while. Smaller quantities raise your self-confidence, your self esteem, as you get thinner and thinner. But if you ever eat more than you wanted with the new eating habits, you're free from guilt or self-punishment, as you simply make up for it by eating less later. A little more here, a little less there, and you're back in balance. Once in a while, you may even plan ahead for a heavier meal by eating little or no food beforehand.

And as your body adjusts to these new eating habits, half way through a meal you begin to notice the full feeling; the body communicates to the mind that it's getting full rather quickly, and the mind makes the logical and reasonable decision to...*stop there*. You push away from the table, and you feel so much better about yourself. You are very happy to simply leave the food and forget about it. There are simply other things you'd rather do or think about.

As you plan your meals at specified times and locations, you'll find it easy to avoid unhealthy snacking, because you know meal time will arrive sooner or later. It will simply be less often that foods cross your mind, so notice how you forget to even think about foods. If you do snack once in a while, you do it with good conscience. As you develop the habit of only eating when you are physically hungry, you only eat just enough healthy food to satisfy your hunger and you're done; you're eating reasonable portions and you've had enough, noticing that most of the day you are free from hunger. And you can go longer periods of time without food, knowing meal times will arrive sooner or later. You simply put your mind on other things. You feel fine with eating less food. With each passing day you notice the difference in the mirror, how the clothes fit, how your body shape is changing back to the way you want it. It's a positive boost to your moral each day knowing you are making progress, so you carry a more positive attitude most of the time.

With the mind and body of a thinner person, you have what you want, need, and desire. You'll be taking care of yourself more—with less food—and feel more satisfied, a higher self image...self control, more self confidence...self assured. The long term stress of weight retention has disappeared now. It's as if a weight has been lifted with a *new you*. The old ball-and-chain effect from dragging around poor eating habits is gone forever, and there's a wonderful feeling of freedom. Take a few moments now to imagine yourself in the very near future as a thinner person and notice how much happier you are...how much better that thinner body feels. (Long Pause.)

WEIGHT LOSS II

You're beginning to notice all of the subtle and positive changes that you are experiencing from hypnotic suggestion and you are more motivated than you've been in a long time to reduce weight, and you're doing it; it's great to be doing it. You are finding things you dislike about fattening foods, avoiding them more often, and you are finding things you like about smaller portions. You are more attracted to healthier-lighter foods. You are enjoying healthier foods more. There are many subtle shifts that are taking place for you subconsciously.

You are on your way as you have started achieving your goals of becoming a happier, thinner, and healthier person. You're moving away from all the past discomforts, the stresses over weight and eating problems. You are removing all negative self-talk about yourself now, and replacing it with positive messages, so you're more relaxed, more relaxed with the whole idea of becoming thinner. Notice how you have shifted your attitude away from problem eating habits and become more positive about healthy eating habits.... because this is what you really want. You want to be thin and satisfied at the same time, and this is what is starting to happen. You're going to be very motivated now to continue to slim down further from here. And you're going to do it the easier way, with healthy, satisfying eating habits; a routine life-style of healthiness.

Remember that this still has nothing to do with dieting or conscious willpower. You have a deeper, subtle, subconscious willpower now that comes from within. Never again will you deprive yourself of food; dieting is just an unpleasant memory from the past and those days are over forever. You have begun to create the eating habits of a thinner person. Your conscious desires now match the subconscious urges to eat like a thin person. (List changes here.)

You've begun to think about foods more logically, you've happily severed any emotional ties to foods, so continue to notice that you forget to even think about many foods; you've put food out of the mind more often and you are only eating when you are physically hungry... only once in a while when you are physically hungry. Lots of types of food are appearing less and less appetizing now. Most of the time, food is simply unimportant. Your snacks are healthier and smaller. You're avoiding fattening foods or junk foods and feeling really good about yourself...you're just glad to be without the stress that heavier foods used to cause you in the past. The truth is, the old, unhappy eating habits are broken and you're experiencing a wonderful feeling of freedom, self control, self accomplishment, self assured. Your self image is higher. You're feeling much better about yourself with all the changes that are allowing you to reach your goals of being a happier, healthier thinner person.

Notice how satisfied you feel with the new eating habits. To your own amazement, you can eat less frequently with smaller portions and be satisfied. You may even begin to test yourself by giving yourself smaller portions than usual just to see how much you can get away with and still feel satisfied. You know in good conscience, you could go back for more, but you simply don't feel like it. You're full. You don't need much anymore, and you feel great. You're feeling more healthy both physically and emotionally. To your own amazement, it will take very little to satisfy yourself now. You are more aware of your choices now. You are making more reasonable choices at the grocery store, restaurants, even at home. You are eating less, and getting more self-esteem, inner control, strength and a higher self image. You're choosing health over the problematic overeating habits of the past. You choose smaller reasonable portions, and you're amazed, as the stomach continues to shrink, getting smaller and smaller, so it gets full quicker. Notice how the full message comes from the body into the mind more quickly, and you're in control now.... you'll be able to stop when you're full, and you are very, very, proud of yourself. There's a new sense of inner-strength, and inner control. Now that you're becoming more and more satisfied with eating less food, notice how the body begins to appear thinner to yourself and others... It's going to be time soon for the positive comments, "Are you losing weight?" they'll say. Whether you're at a social occasion, a restaurant, or at home preparing food for yourself or others, you have your own separate eating habits that make you thinner and happier—and you're still being just as sociable. You feel fine eating around anyone else, and eating less, because your eating habits have nothing to do with other peoples eating habits. It's *your* mind and *your* body that you're taking charge of, so you'll continue to enjoy your personal responsibility to yourself to continue to be happier, thinner, and healthier with these healthy eating habits.

You're using the power of the subconscious mind and its easy to see that you're happier avoiding fattening foods... you're satisfied as a moderate eater. You're experiencing more balance, moderation, and control now, and you're feeling better about this than you have about anything for a long time. Your body--your temple, is now becoming a sacred and honored place for your spirit. You honor your body more. You give it what it needs to sustain a healthy life with physical energy, but it's all in moderation. You're feeling more spiritual now. You're attaining a higher level of spiritual growth with your etheric body blending with your physical body, and it feels wonderful. You're achieving your birthright to have a thinner healthier body now. The long time stress of weight retention has been lifted and there's a new path in your life that is much more satisfying. Take a few moments now to see yourself months into the future as a happier, healthier thinner person. Notice how safe and wonderful it feels to wear that thin body...Notice how good you feel physically... mentally... and emotionally. (Pause, and awaken.)

Weight: Moderation

You're moving into a life-style of balance and moderation. You have many choices that you can make to achieve a healthier state of balance and moderation. You are in control of certain things in your life, and one of them is food. You are self-empowered by the fact that you can control what you eat, and how much you eat. You can achieve more balance and harmony in your life by eating smaller portions of food. You are attracted to the idea of balance and moderation each day, over the things you have power over now, like food. You begin to notice others who have the power, the balance, the harmony in their life because their food intake is under control.... you want to have what they have. Notice their stomach is smaller; they stop eating when they are full. You want this for yourself... you deserve the inner-peace and balance from having a smaller stomach.

You want a smaller stomach and you want to start by eating smaller portions of foods throughout the day. You're going to start noticing when you are getting full, feeling full quicker at meal time. It only takes a small amount of food start feeling full. You only eat when you're hungry, only eating food when you are physically hungry and that is only once in a while. You wait to feel hungry before eating... never again will you eat food when you aren't hungry. Never again will you fill the stomach when it's already full. In good conscience, you may fill the stomach when you are hungry and it's OK. You feel fine eating when you are hungry, but notice, you truly are only hungry once in a while. It's simply less often that food crosses your mind. You are going longer and longer periods of time where food simply doesn't even cross your mind. You are waiting to eat only when you are logically and truly hungry. When you do decide to eat, you are eating moderate portions, choosing moderate portions, knowing in good conscience you could go back for more, but after eating small portions, you're satisfied. You may be amazed sometimes that you are satisfied with smaller portions, but your stomach is full. You don't want any more food. You put your mind on something else. You may even notice that you took too much, so you leave it, you leave it and feel fine, you feel fine leaving it behind. Leaving it makes you feel happier, healthier, you're living more with balance and harmony in yourself, and therefore in other areas of your life as well.

Your stomach is shrinking with smaller portions now; the stomach is getting smaller and you're getting fuller quicker at meal times. You're taking smaller and smaller portions because you know it's taking less food to fill the stomach all the time. Less food, smaller stomach, then less food. As the stomach shrinks you're listening to your stomach, eating slower, getting full quicker, smaller portions again, full quicker, smaller stomach... you're in moderation, harmony, and balance and you feel great just leaving all that food behind. You feel wonderfully satisfied, a wonderful sense of freedom with the smaller stomach and less food. You feel satisfied with less food. You feel great. You look better... You're feeling fine, you are starting to look great. You're getting thinner with each passing day... thinner and happier. There is an inner peace with food in moderation now. There is an inner peace and harmony living life with less food, because you are achieving the life-style of a thinner-happier person.

You're eating less often because there are other things you'd rather do or think about. There are other things you'd rather do or think about other than food. There are other things that are simply more important than foods that you'd rather occupy your mind with. You are more productive, happier, and self-accomplished by forgetting about foods, putting the idea of food or meals out of your mind and becoming a more relaxed, peaceful, and successful person. You simply eat less food, less often. You simply have better things to do and you know that there will be time to eat later. You are achieving moderation and balance in your life. Food is in balance now, so your life becomes a symbol of balance and moderation. You've accomplished moderation, so now your life-style is reflecting moderation mentally, physically as you get thinner and thinner, and emotionally. You arc experiencing more balanced emotions as a result. You have a wonderful self image now. You're reaching moderation and you feel a much more positive self image. Your self esteem is higher and you feel great...looking good.

Weight: Body Image & Appreciation

You are beginning to notice the type of body you want because you are starting to imagine it. You imagine your body healthier and thinner, and this makes you feel better. You like your body image in your mind's-eye this way, so now is the time to begin to imagine the body you want. You imagine a positive body image for yourself. This feels wonderful, to imagine the body you want; thinner, more attractive, more attractive clothes. Your imagination is going to start superimposing upon your body, and this is helping it respond. When you focus your imagination on the body you want, it starts responding.

You'll notice it first responding to positive imagination by imagining what it is going to look like in the mirror. There are some features of your body that you like. There are simply features of your body that you know look attractive and will continue to look more and more attractive as you get thinner, and thinner. You like certain things about your body now, and yet there are areas you are going to imagine differently. You are going to image yourself now with nice hair. You like your hair. You are imagining yourself with a thinner face. You like yourself this way. You are imagining yourself with a more pronounced chin. You like yourself this way. You are imagining yourself with a protruding chest. You like your chest as it protrudes from the front of your body over your stomach. You imagine your stomach shrinking; imagine a smaller stomach. With each passing day it pulls in a little. It gets flatter with each passing day... a little flatter as you keep getting a little happier, more and more content. Imagine the handles simply shrinking. Yes, this is what you really want... the thinner you. Imagine this, the beautiful you underneath it all. You like yourself. You have a thinner more spiritual body underneath it all and your imagination is showing you this because it's true. Now you notice your hips getting smaller; your waistline smaller. Imagine that, a thinner waistline when you look in the mirror. Your clothes fit better. You like yourself more this way. Now imagine your thighs looking thinner. You love your thighs now as you imagine what they will look like. As you're getting thinner, your thighs look more muscular; the outer layer is disappearing and your legs look much better. Your calves, ankles, feet, smaller and more attractive. Imagine you're smaller, more defined, more attractive, and you like yourself this way. You love the way you look. You imagine that you look wonderful now, and your body is responding.

Imagine the ideal body now as you're smoothing over any of the fatty areas with your hands. Rub it off. Rub your hands over those areas so that your body gets the message now... it's time to reshape, redistribute this material. You smooth it away, feeling the thinner you underneath it all.... the real you. You like the real you. Smoothing, thinning, rubbing and your body is responding; it needs to know what you want so it can change. Smoothing away what you don't want anymore, and it's responding. You look at your body the way you want it, caressing the present and future curves. Yes, there is a natural body you are remembering, you are projecting into your future. You're training your body to release the extra and preparing for more and more thinness, naturally positive thinness.

Imagine your self image now, much more positive, carrying yourself differently. You hold your posture different now. You like sitting straight, you like standing straight. You hold your head up higher. You tighten your stomach muscles and straighten your back because you feel better about yourself, who you are, as a thinner person. You're becoming a thinner person and your posture is changing to reflect this. You have a higher self esteem. You like yourself more. You feel better. You're imagining your body as thin and more attractive. You wear more attractive clothes and others are noticing... you're getting thinner. You like yourself. You like the way you look, feel, hold yourself around others. You're more confident. You feel more positive every day. You're satisfied with your body and it continues to respond to your thoughts... thinner... more satisfying. You're happier with yourself on many levels, in mind, body, and spirit. You feel more spiritual as you achieve your ideal body, your natural inborn body that spirit intended for you. You feel more natural imagining your lighter body. Your thinner natural body. You feel fine with this naturally thinner body image. You feel fine.

Weight: Eliminating Excess

There are certain foods that you may be craving and that's okay; it's fine that you're this way, so you are going to accept yourself. Accept that you have preferences for certain foods. You like them and it's OK, you can still create a thinner body with these desires, because you are going to create three alternatives that will always leave you feeling satisfied. You won't be missing a thing, you will experience satisfaction and become a thinner person in the process. So now is the time to tune your subconscious mind so that you get what you want and still create a thinner, happier, healthier body. So now you will need to listen to these three suggestions either consciously or subconsciously:

Number one... You are going to start looking for substitutes that are less fattening and still give you a great amount of satisfaction. You are going to start taste testing and noticing that you still have everything you desire by eating a less fattening substitute. You are seeking and finding less fattening alternatives that leave you feeling satisfied, that leave you feeling thinner, happier, and healthier. You like your new substitute foods just as much now. You train your taste buds to like them and you are getting used to a thinner, healthier, happier food, and you like yourself more. You are getting everything under control with the satisfying substitute food. You feel fine with this, you feel fine.

Number two... OR-You are noticing that if and when you eat your favorite food, regardless of how fattening, you are cutting the quantity down and still feeling satisfied. Notice that you could even eat half the quantity and still be satisfied. You are satisfied with less. You are eating slower, savoring the taste, and you simply need less and less. It's the quality you are after. You hate what the larger quantities do to your body. You like what smaller quantities do... they leave you feeling thin and happier. And to your own amazement, you can have a smaller quantity of your favorite foods and still be satisfied. You've had enough and you feel fine. A little bit less and a lot more self esteem, because you're getting in control. You shave a little off, and you give yourself so much more in having a thinner, happier life-style. Notice that with time you shave a little more from the quantity and you feel fine. You are achieving a balance in your life now, by eating less, but feeling satisfied, completely satisfied. You feel fine with a little less, and you still have what you want, you still have what you need. You feel fine.

Number three... OR- You may decide to completely avoid this problematic food. You are completely against it, because it is the one thing you must eliminate from your life to become a thinner person. So you do it. You give it the ax, because you know that you are the type of person that has to do it this way. You eliminate this problem once and for all from your life. You give it up for now... and then you ask yourself... "How long can I go without it?" It may be days; it may be weeks; it may be months... but you're going without it and focusing on your thinness. You want to be thin much more than overeat this food. You have a burning desire to be thin so you eliminate it. And then, if and when the day comes where you decide to partake in that favorite food again, you go all out... you eat, and eat, and devour this stuff so that you make sure you've had enough. If you ever touch that certain food ever again, you know you will binge on it until you are sick. You know you would do this, so you remove it completely, because you don't want to be sick. Binging makes you feel stuffed and sick. You feel very sick, that overly stuffed feeling and you would hate that food now; you would learn to hate that food, because once you get sick of it, you never have the taste for it again. You never have a taste for it again, because you've had enough; you've had more than enough, so you release it; you let it go. You've had enough to be satisfied for a lifetime. You release it. You release it and it releases you and you have a wonderful sense of freedom. You feel free. You eliminate it again, and you know with good conscience that you could eat too much again, but you don't like that. You don't like overeating anymore. You go back to what's right for you and you find that you have less and less desire for any past favorite foods. Less and less desire. You put them out of your mind and you are free. You are free. You are satisfied without them.

You are free and you like yourself better this way. You have a higher self image, more self esteem. You like engaging in the thinner habits that were suggested, because they are leading to the habits of a thinner person. You have the life-style of a person who's getting thinner and thinner, and you're in control. You're gaining control over your eating habits and noticing other positive changes in your life. You've taken your power back from those substances, and you feel great. You feel self-empowered. You realize now that you are a success. You have mastered one of your greatest challenges in life and never again will any substance dominate you. You are the master of your destiny now that you are in control. You've mastered one problem and now you have more faith in your abilities. You feel as if you can do anything you set your mind to, because your have more control over your eating habits. You have more control, inner strength. You like who you are now. You are putting things in perspective and in moderation and you like who and what you are becoming. You are getting thinner through these choices and you are achieving a balance with this moderation in your life. You're thinner, happier, and healthier and you have an overall positive self image. You're satisfied with your choices to be different, thinner, and you feel fine. You feel great.

Weight: Food Aversion Metaphor

You heard of a very reasonable, all inclusive hotel where the service is impeccable. Included is world renowned room service. For a special treat you've checked yourself in to a nice and comfortable hotel room. You notice your room service menu, and to your own amazement, the menu just happens to have all of your favorite meals, snacks, beverages, and desserts on it. You call down for room service and tell them that you're glad to see that they have all your favorite foods. You list them, and they tell you that they will give you whatever you desire.... you're really excited; it's a special event, only for yourself. You say "yes" to all of the items to be sent over and hang up the phone in anticipation.

After you complete your call, the phone rings again; it's a good friend that you haven't been able to get in touch with for a while. In your excitement you're unaware of room service delivering your order. You barely notice out of the side of your eye that tray after tray begins to be placed in your room. You keep talking, looking forward to your eminent feast, but you're still happy to be catching up and being in contact with your long-time friend.

At some point, you realize that the food service trays are blocking your way to freedom. Tray after tray is piling up and quickly it is all you can see; you tell your friend to hold, so you can put a stop to the misunderstanding with the kitchen. But they're out of control, as your favorite foods are now beginning to become your worst nightmare, blocking your way to freedom. The food is just piling up in a big pile now, as if you are trapped in a landfill of your favorite foods. You look for a way out of your dilemma. You get back to your friend on hold trying to explain your dilemma. They remind you that they warned you that this could happen, and that you were aware of this all along. You ask for their help, but they remind you that you already know what to do about this. The pile of food is now starting to spoil; it starts getting a putrid smell, giving off gases. You realize that every fattening meal that you've ever eaten has been delivered to you room now. You hate the bugs and hatching flies. The decomposing matter from the years of excess is a grim reminder that you have been given chances to change... the chance to change, that you wish you had again.

You want a way out; you look and look. You say to yourself, "There must be a way out." And then you see a light above the pile of food that's pressing against you. You're against the wall, but you can move your feet. You lift one foot after the other, one at a time to step upward, upward onto the pile toward the light. You're bound and determined to reach the top of the pile and you step down on the mush, but you're climbing. You get to where you can see over the top. It's the door. It's open, but un-reachable. You hear your friend's voice beyond the food at the door asking you where to start. He asks you, "What is the one thing to remove that will make the biggest difference for your escape to freedom." You tell your friend what it is, and your friend starts removing the substance that's trapping you. You can see your friend's face now as the food pile becomes reduced. You say to yourself, wait a minute, that's not who you thought it was; this person who's rescuing you is actually your *higher-self*.

You've come to your own rescue. You are in control now. You decide how to remove these things; you've realized that it's time to put a stop to this nonsense, these dichotomies in your life. You decide now to step through that door and leave that mush behind you... behind you forever. And as you step through that door, your higher-self embraces you. You've become one, now. You're one with yourself, removing all inner conflicts with yourself, forever. You're happy because you finally made it. You've done it. You've removed all blockages to your success and you have a new lease on life... a new life-style of freedom, enjoyment, and higher understandings. You're free now.

Weight: Increasing Metabolism & Movement

As you relax further and further you'll begin to mentally shift your metabolism with your imagination. You can choose a metaphor now in your mind's eye that represents increased metabolism. You will be creative now and focus on an image that represents increased metabolism.

Now brighten-up the colors in the mind's eye and notice how much more clear the image appears...

Notice all the details you hear in the image and then turn up the volume so that you may experience these with more detail....

Now, imagine the feelings of increased metabolism. Notice the inward and outward feelings and sensations...

Now take some deep breathes. Inhale and hold a little while... and then exhale... Inhale again with a deep breathe... and then exhale again. Repeat this several times until the sensation of stretching the chest and neck muscles begins to disappear. Inhale... Exhale... Over and over until deep breathing feels relaxing, refreshing, and very natural. As the chest cavity expands, you will notice that inhaling a large amount of air takes less and less effort. Notice how your posture improves from exercising your lungs. You sit straighter, you stand straighter. Your chest protrudes over the rest of the body and you begin to appear thinner. Your body is truly burning up more energy, more excess fatty tissue, as a result of deep, deep, natural breathing. Your metabolism is increasing every day because you are breathing more naturally, more deeply. Your respiration increases with this. As you breathe deeper each day, your heart and lungs are healthier, working with less effort to send oxygen to every cell and tissue in the body. More oxygen, burning more fat, increasing metabolism, remembering to breathe... now, breathe... breathe regularly and deeply, feeling more energetic, like you have more oxygen to your muscles, so you feel like moving around more now. You feel the need for more movement each day.

Notice how you feel like stretching more often, you feel like stretching your joints and muscles more routinely as part of your day, as part of your daily routine. Stretching out all of the stiffness and feeling more positive, more flexible, more agile, more comfortable. You stretch and move around more. You walk more. If you get a chance, you walk instead of ride. You simply and easily feel like going the extra distance. Go the distance. And as you increase your breath, movements and activity each day, you improve the oxygen to the brain, so you begin to think more clearly and remember things more easily. You increase your circulation as you breathe and move, so your brain is more efficient. You think more clearly. You feel thinner, more toned. When you get an opportunity to be more active, to breathe more, to increase metabolism, you take it. Knowing your limitations and exercising your limitations, you come across an opportunity for more movement and you take it. You say, "Yes." It may be when you're alone or you may have the opportunity to join a class. Either way, you find what suits you, what you're capable of and you begin to say, "Yes." And you do it. You just do it. You seize the opportunity to feel better, breathe better and burn off more fatty tissue.

You are happier with more movement, and your body responds by getting thinner. You may start increasing your movement and breathing by taking the long way to your room, your office, your neighbor's, your local shopping areas. You want the activity for your body. You want to have it. Your body wants you to do it. You give that satisfaction, that natural satisfaction to your body now, because you deserve to improve it, tone it, utilize it to the fullest and then relax it. Your body relaxes more deeply afterward. You feel more relaxed, less stressed, you forgot all about stress. You breathe out all your stress. Breathing deeply and relaxing. Breathing deeply and relaxing. You have more energy available and you like yourself more this way. You are more aware of your body's needs and you are satisfying it more often, even if it's just minutes at a time.... you are allowing it to move more, breathe more, and burn up more energy. The body's responding, getting thinner, feeling better, you feel better about yourself with a higher self image. You have more self esteem and it feels great. You feel more balanced in mind, body and spirit. You take care of your physical vehicle now and you have more value in your life. You simply feel good. You like your new metabolic rate and this adjustment. You like it as you shed the weight. You feel great.

Weight. Loss: Choices

Now you are going to become aware of all of your choices... all foods and eating are going to become a conscientious plan, a conscious choice for the better. You are going to become uniquely aware of the type of foods and the quantities of foods that you are choosing to eat in every moment. When a person chooses, now, to become thinner, they are beginning a new-healthier and happier life style, the life-style and habits of a thinner, happier, freer self-accomplished person. Each and every healthier and happier choice begins at the start of each day, and each and every choice for healthier foods leaves yourself thinner, happier, and more satisfied, simply more content and satisfied.

Your positive thinner choices for yourself start at the beginning of each new bright and beautiful day of your new satisfying life. Each choice toward thinness in the morning will lead you to have a happier morning, starting your day off on the right foot; morning choices to choose thinner foods, or smaller amounts of thicker foods, stimulate an inner peace, happiness and freedom within you. If the foods at breakfast are thinner foods, like cereal, fruit, and other grains, you eat a reasonable quantity and leave the table a success. You are a success, because you are very satisfied, very satisfied with healthier breakfasts in reasonable quantities. You are leaving the table a thinner person and there is a feeling of self accomplishment. Your self image is higher when you leave the table having eaten thinner healthier foods. And you're satisfied, you're very satisfied...

And once in a while you will be presented an opportunity to eat thicker foods... foods that in larger quantities could leave you thicker, heavier, and uncomfortable. When thicker foods are presented to you, you lose your appetite for them, even at the sight of thicker foods, you lose your appetite for them. Smelling thicker foods like high-fat meats, eggs, butter, and other greasy foods coat your sensing cells in your nose with grease, from the grease in the air where these things are cooked... and you lose your appetite for these things. Yet, you may notice that if you choose to sample these foods once in a while, you do it guilt-free. You are going to these occasionally when you want to, and you are going to do it guilt free, because you are going to limit your quantities. You will occasionally choose only small amounts of fattening foods and this will set you free. You are completely satisfied with smaller amounts of fattening foods at lunch and at dinner as well, and this gives you an inner strength, a freedom to become the thinner person you deserve to be. And when you leave in the morning, you will be planning for a happier, healthier, thinner you at lunch time...because you may either be packing a healthier lunch that you will take with you to work, or you may be planning to cook a healthier lunch, or you may be planning a healthier lunch at a restaurant. You want to choose a healthier lunch, because you deserve to be a happier, healthier, and thinner person.

Even at lunch breaks, you are making conscientious choices about the types of foods that are right for you, thinner for you, leaving you feeling satisfied. You will be loosing your appetite for thicker foods, eating less, eating slower, feeling satisfied quicker. And you end your lunch break feeling a wonderful sense of freedom. Feeling satisfied with your choices, feeling much better about who you are and where you are headed... a thinner happier life-style.

Many times you may forget about snacking...putting it out of your mind. On the rare occasion if you should ever think about snacking, you will think about making the right choice, healthier snacks, or lower quantities of unhealthy snacks, lower quantities, feeling happier with less.. Avoiding snacking makes you feel better physically and mentally. You feel a more positive attitude by reducing or eliminating snacking, and especially feeling happier with thinner snacking, thinner foods when you do decide to snack... thinner foods, healthier foods, happier, thinner, with a higher self image and self esteem.

At dinner time you choose the healthier, happier and thinner foods; small quantities of the thicker foods. You are making the right choices for yourself. Choosing healthier foods to eat leaves you more satisfied, freer to be who you want to be, thinner, happier. You are choosing smaller quantities especially at dinner time. You choose normal quantities of healthier foods. You cut back but miss nothing. You miss nothing because you are satisfied with your dinner choices. You socialize but you are aware of your best, most happiest choices, and when you make the best and smartest choices you feel good, you feel self accomplished. You feel successful. You leave the table happy with your choices to be thin, and there is a wonderful feeling of freedom.

Your choices start at the grocery store. There, you notice that each healthier choice you make, makes you feel one notch better; it's one step closer to freedom and happiness. You may decide to choose a few thicker foods, but you do it guilt free, because you know that if you partake in the thicker foods, you eat reasonable amounts. The choice for thicker foods may simply be for other people in the family, people you live with may want thicker foods, but you're loosing your appetite for them. You choose more and more healthy foods each time you shop because they are tasting better to you. Healthier foods simply appear more appetizing. Your grocery store shopping is a pleasurable, successful experience, because you leave the store knowing you are a success. You are becoming a thinner person through all of your choices... happier choices at home, when going out, at restaurants, and more.

After dinner, or at night, you choose healthier snacks and are satisfied. Notice, however, you feel like avoiding the kitchen. At night, you want to stay away from the kitchen. You want to only do the right thing. You feel satisfied without food, because your stomach is still full from dinner. You are satisfied without food in the late evening, but you know that if at any time, you physically feel that the body is hungry, in good conscience, once in a while you may choose a happier, healthier food in reasonable quantities. However, you notice that you simply have lost the appetite for food at night. You lost your appetite because you are satisfied without it; happier, freer, healthier, feeling a higher self-esteem in the evenings with your choices to be thin. Satisfying, happier, and much healthier choices each day of your life... and maintaining the happier life-style of a thinner person. You feel great... you're in the habit of healthier daily choices and you feel great.

Your Slender Image

You have been eating much more than your body either needs or wants. And you, the mind, controls eating—not the stomach, not the mouth; no, you, the mind. You are beginning today at this same mind level to program yourself, to develop new habits, and to set new goals. You are laying the mental foundation for the new you, a cheerful and attractive you, the you that you always knew you could be.

Of great importance to this positive new you, to your healthy, active and attractive body, is the fact that the less you eat, the happier you feel. The less you eat, the more you smile. Now the less you eat, the more relaxed you are. Now the less you eat, the better you look. Now the less you eat, the more patience you have.

Now the less you eat, the more motivation you have.

Now the less you eat, the more energy you have.

Now you find satisfaction in eating less. You can pride yourself in knowing that each time you do eat less, you are rewarding your slimmer self: the self you want to be, the slim self you are becoming, the slim self that you *already are* deep within. Whenever you choose this new image of yourself, you experience new feelings of health and well-being. It feels good to feel good about yourself.

The most amazing thing is that each day now, in your eating habits, you are forming new patterns. Each day now it is easier and easier to eat sensibly. You are gaining new strength, and that strength is the ability to eat sensibly. You can eat sensibly and still be satisfied.

As you exercise that new strength, it grows; it becomes more able, more fit. And each day now, as you eat sensibly, this becomes more and more reinforced, more a natural part of your life. It is like using the muscles of your arm. As you use them each day, they become stronger. As you eat sensibly each day, it becomes easier and easier to continue in a practical way, a sensible way.

Eating sensibly means that you mentally ask your own body what foods it needs. Then, quietly listen to your own body, and it will tell you what foods it wants and needs for you to eat sensibly, nutritiously, and happily. Eating sensibly is eating slowly and carefully, always concentrating on chewing, always thinking of that mouthful that you are chewing. Eating sensibly also means drinking sensibly, drinking more fruit and vegetable juices.

As you exercise and eat sensibly, your body will automatically be regulated to the ideal rate for you to become as slim as you wish to be. By using your creative imagination, you can picture yourself as you would like to be. You can create a positive mental image of yourself as exactly the way you want to be, as exactly the way you want to look. Mentally dress yourself in the clothes you'd like to wear. Create a vivid symbol or mental picture and hold it foremost in your mind. (Pause)

You can see yourself increasing your physical activity by fifteen minutes a day. Listen to yourself breathe better as you are regularly doing and enjoying your favorite exercises. See yourself using your new energy in a positive, constructive way. Feel this new energy going throughout your body, building a healthy new you. Feel how it feels to be slim, trim, and healthy.

You can picture your own bathroom scale or any scale and mentally place upon the scale the exact amount you intend to weigh. (Pause) Just imagine that it has already happened, that you already weigh this amount, that you have already increased your physical activity, that you already look the way you once wished you could look. At one level, you already are this positive you, and you are *really* proud of the results—the way you look and feel.

As you think healthy, you become healthy. Health is an important part of the new you. Breathe clean air, eat sensible food, experience normal daily eliminations, and keep active. Later, when you open your eyes, your inner mind will know that you no longer have to overeat, and you no longer have to be hungry because, when you think of something to eat and it isn't mealtime, then your mind immediately reminds you of something better, more enjoyable, that you can just as easily do. It can be whatever you wish, something that really satisfies you.

You can enjoy whatever you do, even if it is by yourself. You can find yourself enjoyable. You can find yourself good company. You can find yourself fun to be with. As you tune in to yourself, you can understand yourself, you can love yourself. You can have a positive conversation with yourself, laugh and joke with yourself. Sing and dance with yourself. The more you learn to love yourself, the easier it becomes to develop positive change in your life.

You are developing a new attitude, for you are what you think; and all that you are thinking, you are becoming. Think how happy you are as you become more slim, more healthy every day. You have developed a slim life style. Other people are telling you how good you look, and you really enjoy preparing your food with love and a positive attitude.

Oral Tobacco Cessation I

(**Protective Suggestions**): Every way you do hypnosis is the right way, automatically; If it seems like you've fallen asleep, it's a hypnotic sleep, the subconscious mind still hears all suggestions, and any outside noises will help you relax even further.

Creating the habits of a tobacco-free person is something you're doing for yourself. We are using the power of your subconscious mind, as we place your conscious desires into it; so you're eliminating inner conflicts now, and reaching greater harmony, as your subconscious messages will work in alignment with your conscious desires to be free from tobacco. Your mind will work like one powerful unit geared toward a healthy powerful change. By using the recording and doing hypnosis, you'll be more relaxed each day, making it easier to release this, and you're able to think more clearly, having logical-keener insights. And because of this, you're able to notice realizations of why *you* are becoming an ex (rubber/chewer). You don't care what anybody thinks or what anybody else is doing around you, whether they (rub/chew) or not, because this is something you're *doing for yourself.*

Deep inside you, the reasons you want to become a non-(rubber/chewer) are moving up toward the surface of your mind now—moving up into your awareness. You've been thinking about them for a long time; the deep-down reasons—some of them may even be different than you thought—but they're surfacing. And as they start to surface, you can sense a little growing feeling of anger or irritation from all the things (rubbing/chewing) has done to you over the years...

Slowing you down, all the hassles, health worries, future health concerns for the mouth and stomach, making you feel bad about yourself, premature signs of aging, damaging the body tissues, problems with self image, guilt, self blame, feeling self-conscious and out of control... You know them all better than anyone else. Notice the breathing change as all of the subconscious feelings of irritation and frustration begin to grow toward the (rubbing/chewing) habit itself. I'm just a mirroring these truths back to your mind now...reflecting many of your own thoughts. The truth is that you're *sick and tired* of being controlled by (snuff/chewing tobacco) for so many years. As all the reasons to quit surface in your mind, it's as if there's a smirky smile sneering at you on each (can/pouch) saying, "Do what you're told slave. I'm in control of your life."

But you say, "No. Not anymore." Now you've reached a point where you put your foot down once-and-for-all to erase this problem out of your life. It's as if there's a brown gooey CD or tape coated with tar and chemicals in the back of your mind labeled, "reasons for (rubbing/chewing)". Your subconscious mind has been playing this over-and-over to yourself for such a long time. Because it has all the false reasons like; looking sophisticated, sexy, young, stress-reduction and other lies on it, I want you to pull the bad-habit tape or CD out of your mind, put it into a cassette tape or CD player and jam down the red erase button to erase all the years of lies and as they spin away the only thing left of this dirty habit is the *smell of manure* (pause).

Now notice, regardless of the mood, stresses, ups and downs through the natural course of living life, you'll continue to remain an ex (rubber/chewer). Whether you're by yourself or around others, you're free, once and for all, from this thing and it feels wonderful. You feel much better quitting this thing, and you're more relaxed everyday because you're free from the stress that it used to cause you for such a long time. Notice, how you find that you even enjoy being tobacco free. You like being without it. You like yourself more this way. And as you think back on all the frustration you experienced, you realize it had nothing to do with the good person you are.

Now you're reaching an awareness—that (rubbing/chewing) has *nothing to do* with boredom, meals, drinking, stress, sex, fears, worries over others, anger or frustrations with people or situations. (Rubbing/chewing) with machines like radios, telephones, TVs, and automobiles is kids stuff; and socializing with peer-pressure friends, or hiding it from authority figures like parents is unnecessary now. You're older and wiser now. You are looking at this in a different light. You have shifted your attitude to where you don't want to do this unhealthy thing anymore.

The idea of (rubbing/chewing) is really dull, it's boring. It's like doing chores or paying the bills, and if you can be without one bill you've been paying with your health, why not? The truth is, (snuff/chews) have nothing to do with the way you feel. You're eating habits remain unaffected because you're simply returning back toward a normal inborn state of being....for example, a baby is born without tobacco juice in its mouth. You'll have the health you had before you ever started (rubbing/chewing)—this is the mind and body of a tobacco-free person.

You feel so free without tobacco, you feel just fine without (snuff/chews). You feel satisfied with the life-style of a tobacco-free person. It's a wonderful life without tobacco. You've seen others do it. You know of others who have quit successfully, and you know that you can do it too. You feel great without (snuff/chews) each and every day, from this day forward.

Now, there are two things you need to be aware of either consciously or subconsciously:

#1) You're going through a period of change, and in the short term, the thought of (rubbing/chewing) may cross your mind. If it does, it's simply considered a *brief memory from the past* . The mind is like a TV screen and now you're in control of the channel. Notice how quickly the channel changes to something you would rather do or think about, and you forget to even think about it. You forget to even think about it.

#2) An urge or craving is physically impossible. Those thoughts are fleeting memories now, and the serious thought of a (rub/chew) will almost always bring back bad memories of this dirty habit. But remember, brief memories of the old habit disappear as quickly as a breath of fresh air.

Now as you've become tobacco-free, the thought of (rubbing/chewing) again would be like pouring a saliva cup down your throat, burning, sick, and dizzy—just like the first time. But you're free from the need to test yourself because you may think back and say, "I've had enough trouble from this." And now that you are focusing on other things that you'd rather do or think about, it's almost as if you've never been a (rubber/chewer) in the first place. You forget to even think about it.

Notice how satisfied you are without (snuff/chews)—feeling that you still have everything you need. As an ex-(rubber/chewer), you have all the rewards and excitement that you want. You're without tobacco, and you relax just as quickly and easily. You're feeling really good about this, you feel better without it now. Because of this, you'll do whatever it takes to assure your success. Now there's something new... more control, inner-strength, self confidence, self assured, a feeling of self-accomplishment, with more faith in your health and longevity. It feels as if a weight has been lifted—a new you. The old ball-and-chain effect of being tied to a dirty habit is gone, and there's a wonderful feeling of freedom. You feel great; you feel just fine without tobacco. You prefer the tobacco-free life-style this day, and every day for the rest of your life. It's a wonderful way to live your life.

Everything will seem a little easier and more enjoyable. You're going to be successful, so the future is very bright...Imagine yourself as a tobacco-free person now within the next few moments and notice that you're feeling fine, you're relaxed; you're at peace with yourself, you're much happier, healthier, and freer to be who you want to be (pause).

Oral Tobacco Cessation II

Note:
At client interview, focus on positive results—the amount of (rubbing/chewing) they don't do anymore. Give credit where it is deserved, "Congratulations", "You're successful; I'm sure you're going to maximize whatever success you've had from here" etc...

Suggestions:
The purpose of this session is to help you adjust to the fact that you're (virtually or permanently) an ex-rubber. With all the changes that have taken place, notice how rewarding it is to be living your life without (snuff/chewing tobacco).

You're very satisfied as a snuff-free person. You feel like you have everything you need or want as an ex-rubber, and you're very proud of yourself. *(If there's a few (rubs/chews) that have been hanging on, relax, they'll fade away rather quickly from here until they're completely gone.)*

You now have the mind and therefore the body of a non-rubber. You're getting more and more healthy with each passing day because hypnosis washes the resins and toxins out of the body more quickly, the circulation improves. You have more oxygen and nutrients going to your brain and muscles so you'll continue to think clearer and feel better. You're reaching your goals of being a (rub/chew-free) person, such as: breathing easier, becoming more active, looking forward to your plans for a longer-happier life, feeling better about yourself, having more time and freedom to do the things that you enjoy in life.

You wouldn't even think twice about picking up the habit with all its problems ever again. With the help of hypnosis, you've erased the habit with all of its worries and problems out of your life and you're able to think about it more logically. You're more realistic as to all the lies and false reasoning that were subconsciously behind it. You're aware of all the changes that have taken place and once and for all you're free from the ongoing hassles and stresses of an old dirty habit. There's a wonderful feeling of freedom. As you've seen for yourself, regardless of the type of day you've had, the stresses, good moods, bad moods, it has nothing to do with (snuff/chewing tobacco). You now have the mind and body of a (non-rubber/chewer). Regardless if you're at work, at home, going out places, socializing, you could care less about (rubbing/chewing). You can be around others who (rub/chew) or even alone, and to your own amazement you're relaxing the natural way—without tobacco.

It's as if you've never (rubbed/chewed) in the first place. The healing forces of the body will get stronger with each passing day as an (ex-rubber/chewer)...it's repairing, restoring, rebuilding, resting and getting healthier quicker. Because you're a clearer logical thinker with the mind and body of a non-rubber each day of your life, it's as if you've gotten your tonsils taken out. When the habit's removed, it's simply gone—permanently...and you have so much to look forward to with the new you...self assured, self accomplished, control, strength—a higher self image and an overall feeling of success. You're a little more relaxed everyday because you're free once-and-for-all from all the problems and stresses that oral tobacco used to cause you in the past. Take a few moments now to see yourself as a happy, healthier (rub/chew-free) person years into the future...notice how good it feels inside, physically, mentally, and emotionally as you wear that wonderfully healthy body.

Smoking Cessation I

Every way you do hypnosis is the right way, automatically; if it seems like you've fallen asleep, it's a hypnotic sleep, the subconscious mind still hears all suggestions; and any outside noises will help you relax even further. Creating the habits of a nonsmoker is something you're doing for yourself. You're using the power of your own subconscious mind, as we place your conscious desires into it; so you're free from the inner arguments with yourself, and you'll take most of the credit. I'm just serving as a guide on a backpacking trip—showing you the way; you're still carrying your own backpack through this change, making the right conscious choices at the right times. By using the recording and doing hypnosis, you'll be able to think more clearly with more logical, keener insights...more realistic. Because of this, you're able to see realizations of why *you* are becoming a nonsmoker. The heck with the people around you, you don't care what they're doing or what they think. This is something you're *doing for yourself.*

Deep inside you, the reasons you want to become a nonsmoker are moving up toward the surface of your mind now—moving up into your awareness. You've been thinking about them for a long time; the deep-down reasons; some of them may even be different than you thought, but they're surfacing. And as they start to surface, you can sense a little growing feeling of anger or irritation from all the things smoking has done to you over the years:

Slowing you down, all the hassles, making you feel bad about yourself, premature signs of aging, damaging the body, problems with self image, guilt and self blame, feeling self conscious and out of control... You know them all better than anyone else. Notice the breathing change as all of the subconscious feelings of irritation and frustration begin to grow toward the smoking habit itself. Not because of what I'm saying; I'm just a mirror of your own mind now—reflecting your own thoughts. You're *sick and tired* of being controlled by (cigarettes) for so many years. As all the reasons surface in your mind, it's as if there's a smirky smile sneering at you on each (cigarette) saying, "Do what you're told slave"...

But now you've reached a point where you put your foot down once-and-for-all to erase this problem out of your life. It's as if there's a black-charred cassette tape or CD coated with tar and chemicals in the back of your mind labeled, "reasons for smoking." You've been playing this over and over to yourself for too long of a time. Because it has all the false reasons on it like, looking sophisticated, sexy, young, and other lies on it, I want you to pull the bad-habit tape or CD out of your mind, put it into a tape or CD player and jam down the red erase button to erase all the years of lies and as they spin away the only thing left of the habit is the *smell of burning plastic.* (pause) {Note: The next paragraph is for spiritually inclined clients}...

You have a new lease on life now, a greater spiritual momentum that spirit has given you to extend and improve your life. You cherish and respect your physical vehicle that the creator made, and now you are willing to treat this temple with respect and only give it healthy air. You will only give it the air that God intended for your lungs, fresh oxygenated air that you were born to breathe.

Notice that regardless of the mood, stresses, ups and downs through the natural course of life you'll continue to remain a nonsmoker. Whether you're by yourself or around others, you're free from all the hassles of lingering thoughts of urges or cravings as they have been extinguished like a chemical fire. You're more relaxed everyday because you're free from the stress that the hundreds of inhaled chemicals have been causing you for such a long time. Notice, how you find that you even *enjoy* being a nonsmoker. And as you think back on all the problems and frustrations smoking used to cause you, you realize it had nothing to do with the good person you are. You simply feel more and more positive and grateful that you are moving past this block in your life now.

Now you're reaching an awareness...that smoking has *nothing to do* with boredom, meals, drinking, stress, sex, fears, worries over others, anger or frustrations with people or situations. Smoking with machines like radios, telephones, TVs, and automobiles is kids stuff; and socializing with peer-pressure friends, or hiding it from authority figures like parents is immature. You are much wiser now from having been a smoker, and now you are exercising your right to live the life you want...living life as a nonsmoker.

The idea of smoking is really dull, it's boring. It's like doing chores or paying the bills, and if you can be without one more bill you've been paying, why not? The truth is, (cigarettes) have nothing to do with the way you feel. Burning leaves & paper are *totally unrelated* to emotions or life's natural course of ups and downs. Your desire for food remains the same or lessens. Your eating habits remain unaffected because you're simply returning back toward a normal state of being. It's impossible to replace something that was never meant to be part of this life in the first place. For example, a baby is born without burning leaves and paper in its mouth. As your body returns back to a healthy state, you'll have the health you had before you ever started smoking — the mind and body of a nonsmoker.

So as you're enjoying a smoke-free life, you'll *absolutely refuse* to let anybody affect your decision to be a nonsmoker — *despite* what anyone else says or does. It's your life, your mind, and your body; the choice to become a nonsmoker was *your* decision...to make yourself happier.

Now, there are two things you need to be aware of either consciously or subconsciously:

#1) You're going through a period of change, and in the short term, the thought of a cigarette may cross your mind. If it does, it's simply considered a *brief memory from the past* . The mind is like a TV screen and now you're in control of the channel. Notice how quickly the channel changes to something you would rather do or think about, and you forget to even think about cigarettes.

#2) An urge or craving is physically impossible. Those thoughts are fleeting memories now, and the serious thought of a (cigarette) will always bring back bad memories around the smoking habit. But remember, brief memories of the old bad habit disappear as quickly as a breath of fresh smoke-free air.

Now as you've become a nonsmoker, the thought of smoking again would be like pouring an ash tray with lit (cigarette) butts down your throat...burning, sick, and dizzy — just like the first time; but you're free from the need to test yourself, because you may think back and say, "Haven't I put myself through enough misery?" With all the lies and false reasons being erased out of the mind, it's almost as if you've never been a smoker in the first place.

Notice how satisfied you are without (cigarettes) — feeling that you still have everything you need. As a nonsmoker, you have all the rewards and excitement that you want, and as a nonsmoker you relax just as quickly and easily. You're feeling better about this than you have anything for a long time. Because of this, you will eliminate any obstacles in the way of your success. Now there's something new... more control, strength, self confidence, self assured, a feeling of self-accomplishment. It feels as if a weight has been lifted — a new you. The old ball-and-chain effect of being tied to a dirty habit is gone forever, and there's a wonderful feeling of freedom.

Everything will seem a little easier and more enjoyable. You're going to be successful, so the future is very bright...Imagine yourself as a nonsmoker in the future, within the next few moments, and notice that you're much happier and healthier...living the life you want. (pause)

Awakening Procedures — (choice to awaken or fall into natural sleep for awaken to the CD/tape) 5...4- Very satisfied as a nonsmoker. 3...2...1

Smoking Cessation II

Note:
During client interview, focus on positive results—the amount of (cigarettes) they haven't smoked. Give credit where it is deserved, "Congratulations", "You're doing great; I'm sure you'll continue to maximize your successes from here" etc...

Suggestions:
The purpose of this session is to help you adjust to the fact that you're (virtually or permanently) a nonsmoker. With all the changes that have taken place, notice how rewarding it is to be living your life without (cigarettes). You have the life that spirit intended for you and your temple, your body, is now being honored in a very respectful way. You like taking care of your physical vehicle more as it promises to help you maximize your health and extend your life.

You're very satisfied as a smoke-free person. You feel like you have everything you need or want as a nonsmoker, and you're very proud of yourself. *(If there's a few (cigarettes) that have been hanging on, relax, they'll fade away rather quickly from here until they're completely gone.)*

You now have the mind and therefore the body of a nonsmoker. You're getting more and more healthy with each passing day because hypnosis washes the resins and toxins out of the body more quickly, the circulation improves. You have more oxygen and nutrients going to your brain and muscles so you'll continue to think clearer and feel better. You're reaching your goals of being a smoke-free person, such as: breathing easier, becoming more active, looking forward to your plans for a longer-happier life, feeling better about yourself, having more time and freedom to do the things that you enjoy in life.

You wouldn't even think twice about picking up the problematic habit with all of its troubles ever again. With the help of hypnosis, you've erased the habit with all of its worries out of your life and you're able to think about it more logically. The hundreds of chemicals that clouded your thoughts about this in the past are no longer present. You're living the life God intended for you in mind, body, and spirit. You're more realistic as to all the false reasoning that was subconsciously behind smoking. You're aware of all the changes that have already taken place and once and for all you're free, free to enjoy your life the natural way. You have more health, money, and now you can actually begin to clearly imagine, perceive, and conceive a longer-healthier life that is more enjoyable. There's a wonderful feeling of freedom. As you've seen for yourself, regardless of the type of day you've had, the stresses, or the ups and downs from living the course of human life, it has nothing to do with (cigarettes). You now have the mind and body of a nonsmoker. Regardless if you're at work, at home, going out places, socializing, you could care less about smoking. You can be around others who smoke or even alone, and to your own amazement you're relaxing the natural way—without cigarettes. You feel very proud of yourself.

It's as if you've never been a smoker in the first place. The healing forces of the body will get stronger with each passing day as a nonsmoker...it's repairing, restoring, rebuilding, resting and getting healthier quicker. You may start feeling a higher presence in your life with a higher connection to spirit, now that this block has been removed. Because you're a clearer logical thinker with the mind and body of a nonsmoker each day of your life, it's as if you've gotten your tonsils taken out. When the habit's removed, it's simply gone—permanently...and you have so much to look forward to with the new you...self assured, self accomplished, control, strength—a higher self image and an overall feeling of success. You're a little more relaxed everyday because you're free once-and-for-all from all the problems and stresses that (cigarettes) used to cause you in the past. Take a few moments now to see yourself as a happy, healthier smoke-free person years into the future...notice how good it feels inside, physically, mentally, and emotionally as you wear that wonderfully healthy body.

Cigarette Cessation

Like a skilled physician, my mind knows the exact remedies I need for a totally healthful way of life. My subconscious mind possesses an inner self-correcting system that is activating right now to realign past patterns and reshape my future. By choosing and developing healthful goals and through clear thinking, I begin a new life, setting new objectives and, with amazing momentum, moving in these directions. I am starting a new life, determined to live each day fully to the utmost of my ability. I have new health and strength and energy to live fully and enjoy everything around me. I feel better and breathe easier. Friends notice the difference and tell me that I look better.

If there are signs of tension, I can relax by taking a deep breath and repeating these words in my mind: "I am relaxed. I am in complete control." I feel better every day because I am living in a new way, with full health and full enjoyment. Each and every day I am doing my best to fulfill my ideals and the purposes of my life, fulfilling them for myself and for everyone I love. As I live fully, smoking becomes less and less a concern. If I think of cigarettes or if someone offers me one, or if I smell the smoke or there is any association with them, I will hear clearly in the back of my mind: "Stop!" I will hear it very strong. It will echo in my mind, "Stop," and I will take a deep breath.

My subconscious mind has far more resources than my conscious mind realizes. My body is now neutralizing the chemicals of the smoke. Even if I try to have a cigarette, my body may reject it. If someone tries to offer me a cigarette, I answer simply, "No, thank you." If I happen to be around people smoking and the smoke annoys me, I put up a mental plexiglass barrier to shield myself. In this way, others' smoke does not bother me or upset my health and well-being. In my mind I hear the words, "I am calm, I am relaxed."

Now I breathe easier and my breath is fresher. I am a clean air person, and I feel new strength and health and vitality. I find new creative outlets for my time and energy—perhaps a hobby or walking in nature or running—whatever I *enjoy* doing. In my creative imagination I visualize a huge blackboard upon which I see the word "cigarettes." I now go to this blackboard and, as I erase that word, I erase, cancel and completely wipe away cigarettes from my life. I have eliminated the need or desire to smoke. (Pause) Now I have a clean slate. I return to the blackboard, pick up the chalk, and in place of the word "cigarettes" I write in capital letters the word "SUCCESS."

The right image comes to my mind as I create a positive symbol, an emblem of my success. I plant a new message in my inner mind, filling it with positive emotion and strength. My goal-image can be whatever I want it to be, and I bring my goals and ideals together into this vivid symbol. (Pause) In a little while when my eyes open, I will be wide awake and comfortable. When I get up from my chair, I will know the joy and vitality of being a nonsmoker and enjoy the feeling of feeling better. My lungs have already started rebuilding. I mentally progress myself forward in time, imagining myself ahead into time—days, weeks, months, and years. What a wonderful feeling of accomplishment. It is accomplished—there was no withdrawal, no nervousness nor anxiety. I walk more, breathe better, and feel healthier. I did a great job—it's *already* accomplished.

Habit Metaphor
mountain traveler

Imagine a traveler who moved out of the hustles and bustles of the city (with all its smog and pollution) and built a home on the lower part of a mountain. The traveler began to take walks out into the forest each day further and further—until one day they looked out the back window of their home and decided that it was time to climb the mountain. The traveler had been thinking about it for a long time and made a choice that this was the time to do it, so the traveler went out and purchased a backpack, brought it home and filled it with all the things that were important in life. The backpack was very full, none the less the (he/she) put it upon (his/her) shoulders, went out and found a trail that other travelers had taken before.

Walking along the path (he/she) began to notice the beauty of all the wild life...the sun shone through the trees to create different patterns of sunlight upon the ground. As the wind blew, the leaves of the trees clattered together to create a natural type of song. There were many types of plants and colorful wild flowers. There was a feeling of being motivated and stimulated to make the climb so the traveler walked forward with a determined pace, and later crossed many fresh water streams and rivers. Sometimes there were bridges provided, and other times the traveler figured out and created ways to cross them by (himself/herself).

A little more than half way up the mountain there was a landing where the traveler took the backpack off of (his/her) shoulders, opened it up, and pulled out all of the things that (he/she) chose to get rid of. After putting them in a trash receptacle there, the traveler decided to forget about them forever. This traveler really didn't care what happened to them, because when the backpack was lifted upon (his/her) shoulders again it felt much lighter. It felt healthier to be able to breathe so much easier. It felt so invigorating that the traveler knew, indeed that (he/she) would reach the top of the mountain.

So as (he/she) continued to walk the path they looked off to one side where (he/she) heard a waterfall in the distance. The traveler thought that perhaps it would be more difficult to create (his/her) own path, but much more rewarding. So the traveler began to chop (his/her) way through the vines and trees until (he/she) reached the beautiful waterfall ...As the sun shone down and reflected in the water, there was a mist that fell upon (his/her) face, which felt cool and refreshing. The birds were singing as they bathed and drank within the puddles that fell upon the rocks at the sides of the waterfall. The traveler went up to taste some of the best tasting spring water they ever had.

After feeling refreshed, the traveler followed the stream to the peak of the mountain where it got much steeper. (He/She) began to pull (himself/herself) up by grabbing at the rocks and vines and indeed the traveler did reach the top of the mountain where there was a wonderful feeling of success, self-accomplishment, health and prosperity. (He/She) looked down into the crease of the mountains where a river flowed. There was a gentle breeze, and (he/she) could hear the various wild-animal sounds, some near, some far away. And as the clouds drifted gently across the sky, the sun was shining down through the clouds and casting different patterns of sunlight upon the various groups of trees on mountain sides.

The traveler sat and pondered many things within (his/her) life, with which (he/she) seemed to reach at least a temporary solution. Appreciating the things surrounding (him/her) in nature and feeling a part of the natural things in life, the traveler knew that (he/she) could return to this special relaxing place in their mind any time (he/she) wanted just by taking the time out to think about it...relaxing naturally with pleasant thoughts. And as the sun began to set over the mountains, they saw one of the most colorful sunsets that anybody had ever seen on the earth.

As it was approaching dusk, it was a signal to return home to take this successfully and naturally-relaxing experience with all the changes into their daily life. The traveler then began walking down the mountain as it was an easy down hill walk. When (he/she) returned home that evening the traveler lied down in the bed feeling naturally exhausted, as (his/her) body melted and soaked deep into the mattress and (his/her) mind drifted off into a deep-distant direction of deep sleep.

Attractive Fingernails

Imagine yourself in the future—progressing through time, moving into time and through time. . . and visualize your hands. . . not as they *used* to be, but as they are *becoming*, as they *are*. Create a vivid image of your fingernails as smooth, attractive (good-looking), and feeling good. Look at them, touch them. Enjoy the way they look and feel. Your mind creates your own reality. And, as your mind is creating this reality for you. . . this is how your hands got better. . .

Long ago, you reached a decision, you made up your mind to the fact that you would like to do something better than bite your nails.

Nobody wants to chew on parts of the body, and you don't have to do anything you don't like.

Your mind is not a computer, but the human mind functions like a computer in many ways. Over the course of time, certain responses get programmed into it. Now your mind is programing in another response. . . a better way of doing things. Whenever it seems you want to bite your nails, your hand will move toward your face, but you can let it stop before it reaches your mouth.

And you will look at your hand— while you decide deliberately— whether you really want to bite your nails. If you decide that you do, then go ahead and chew them. But, of course, nobody really wants to chew on parts of (his/her) own body. So you will decide that you would rather leave your nails alone, and you can let your hand move easily away from your face. And, as you do this, you can remind yourself of how attractive (good-looking) your hands are getting each day.

Day by day, they become more and more attractive. And you become prouder of them as each day passes.

Now, let your mind rehearse this reality for you. Imagine that your hand is moving toward your face. . . without even thinking of it. . . now watch your hand stop. *Really.* . .watch your hand stop.

You're looking at it. . . deciding what you want to do with it. Now, let your hand move away. . . while you remember how attractive your hands are becoming. Each time you do this your programing becomes stronger. And in time. . .any time you choose. . . it will be second nature, and you will remind yourself that you have something better to do with your hands. Something that you choose, the right image, will come to you. Create a vivid goal-image, a symbol of something you really want to do. (Pause) And see it already accomplished, a positive end result, and you are pleased and thankful for your success.

Cancer Recovery (General)

Now one of the things you will train your subconscious mind to do in the days ahead is how to release the stress, anxiety, and fear you have associated with the cancer and to allow the various therapies you are undergoing to be successful. By doing this, you will greatly enhance their effectiveness. You will become relaxed and in balance with the world around you and will let go of all anger and fear associated with your condition. As you become more and more relaxed you will have the strength and confidence to reach the goal you have set for yourself to be cancer-free. Your body will work to kill and eliminate any cancer cells by allowing the therapies to be very effective. As you follow the therapeutic protocols, all healthy cells will be protected by a special coating, while all cancer cells anywhere in your body will be hypersensitive and will be killed off. Not a single cancer cell will survive. Your immune system is greatly enhanced and will help your body to eliminate and kill all cancer cells still present, if any, today and in the future, forever. Your love and acceptance of your own strength will allow you to mobilize your natural healing process to recover quickly and completely from all therapy.

Now you know that this is a time for recovery and healing. The more you allow your mind and body to relax, the more rapidly and completely the recovery and healing will be. You can now allow yourself to permit your body to nurture itself and adjust and thus come into balance to enhance your body's natural healing process. Your desire to recover, heal, and return to a normal life enables you to gain the inner strength and energy within you to meet your goals. You have much to give and much to accomplish in your life. As you participate in your therapies, your ability to relax will enhance the healing process and receptivity to the words of your care-givers and loved ones. They will be speaking to you and their words will be easily understood by you to enhance your healing process and your body's acceptance of the treatments you are undergoing.

Now as you listen to the relaxing sound of my voice, realize that you have the ability to release all cares, fears, worries, or other negative thinking. Right now all your cares, fears, worries, and negative thinking will just drift away. Now I want you to imagine that you are near a large body of water. You may hear the water as it splashes against the shore. You may feel the coolness of a soft breeze off the water as it blows against your skin. You notice a boat nearby. Now I want you to put your thoughts and feelings of self-doubt, being scared, your excessive worry about the cancer, feelings of helplessness, being overwhelmed, not believing in yourself and feelings of frustration on that boat; and allow it to drift off into the distance, off farther and farther away; so far and so distant that you can barely notice it. Allow it to be just a dot on the horizon. However, you do not let the boat totally disappear because you may choose to retain these feelings and retrieve them if you need them. You can always bring the BOAT back. But right now you have no need for these feelings. As you let them go, you gain a sense of peace and calm flowing within your body.

You can now allow yourself the pleasure of watching those feelings drift further and further away into the horizon. Notice that you do not allow them to entirely disappear, so that if you want those feelings back, they will be there. But right now, you have no need for those feelings, so allow them to go off towards the horizon.

Now you are achieving a peaceful, calm attitude with no anger or fear of the future. You move instead to the acceptance and continuation of life. You may want to make changes in your life in the weeks or months ahead and this is wonderful, but for today you are focused only on being healed and happy and relaxed, fully accepting of the love of God, your family and others who love you deeply.

Each day as you listen to this recording, you reaccept the suggestions that are included in this exercise. They are becoming more and more a part of you. Even though you may not consciously remember all of them, they will remain within your subconscious mind and will continue to be more effective than ever before. You will permit yourself to accept the suggestions in this exercise because you want to be cancer-free. And because you want to feel stronger, more in control, relaxed, healthier, and more vigorous. Your desire to be cancer-free, to be strong, and to take control of your life is so great that it easily allows you to accept the suggestions.

Each time you do this exercise, you will feel more alert, refreshed and relaxed, calm, bright, sharp, physically better, emotionally better, mentally better, and spiritually better than you have felt in a long time. These feelings of well-being will remain with you longer and longer with each time you listen to this recording. You truly feel more positive about yourself and the world in which you live. You look at things with a greater amount of faith that everything has a reason, and it will all work out in the end and you will be cancer-free. You feel a higher force, a spiritual force, at work in your life, which facilitates and supports the faith you have. You make a difference in the areas you can, and release the rest. You feel more relaxed in each and every way. You feel wonderful now, self-empowered, more in control. Everything is working out more naturally during the course of your life now and you are able to see yourself cancer-free, participating in all the activities you enjoy. You're living more peacefully and naturally and are more relaxed than ever before. Now take a moment to feel and visualize yourself happy, content, at peace with life with a perfect cancer-free body.

Cancer Recovery: Radiation/Chemotherapy Enhancement

Now one of the things you will train your subconscious mind to do in the days ahead is how to release the stress, anxiety, and fear you have associated with the cancer and to allow the radiation therapy to be successful. By doing this, you will enhance the effectiveness of the radiation therapy which you are undergoing. You will become relaxed and in balanced with the world around you and will let go of all anger and fear associated with your condition. As you are more and more relaxed you will have the strength and confidence to reach the goal you have set for yourself to be cancer-free. Your body will work to kill and eliminate any cancer cells by allowing the radiation therapy to be very effective. As the radiation is absorbed into your body, all healthy cells will be protected by a special coating, while all cancer cells anywhere in your body will be hypersensitive to the radiation and will be killed off. Not a single cancer cell will survive. Your immune system is greatly enhanced and will help your body to eliminate and kill all cancer cells still present, if any, today and in the future, forever. Your love and acceptance of your own strength will allow you to mobilize your natural healing process to recover quickly from all therapy.

Now you know that the time at home and in the hospital is for recovery and healing. The more you allow your mind and body to relax, the more rapidly the complete recovery and healing will be. You can now allow yourself to permit your body to nurture itself and adjust and thus come into balance to enhance your body's natural healing process. Your desire to recover, heal, and return to an active life enables you to gain the inner strength and energy within you to meet your goals. As you have your radiation treatment, your relaxation will enhance the healing process and receptivity to the words of your doctor and the radiation technicians. They will be speaking to you and their words will be easily understood by you to enhance your healing process and your body's acceptance of the radiation.

Now as you listen to the relaxing sound of my voice, realize that you have released all cares, fears, worries, or other negative thinking. Right now all your cares, fears, worries, and negative thinking will just drift away. Now I want you to imagine that you are near a large body of water. You notice a BOAT nearby. Now I want you to put your thoughts and feelings of self-doubt, being scared, your excessive worry about the cancer, feelings of helplessness, being overwhelmed, not believing in yourself, and feelings of frustration on that boat and allow it to drift off into the distance, off further and further away; so far and so distant that you barely notice it. Allow it to be just a dot on the horizon. However, you do not let the boat totally disappear because you may choose to retain these feelings and retrieve them if you need them. But right now you have no need for them. As you let them go, you gain a sense of peace and calm flowing within your body.

You can now allow yourself the pleasure of watching those feelings drift further and further away into the horizon. Notice that you do not allow them to entirely disappear, so that if you want those feelings, they will be there. But right now, you have no need for those feelings, so allow them to go off towards the horizon. These feeling will be there if you want them back or want to be in touch with them.

Now as you enter the place in the hospital where they will do the radiation therapy and are sitting or lying down waiting for the therapy to begin, you can permit your body to become very relaxed by simply closing your eyes and taking a very deep breath, which will cause you to immediately become very relaxed and give you a peace of mind that the therapy will be very effective. It is possible that there may be other noises in the area. These noises will not disturb you; instead they will simply act as a signal to deepen your relaxation and receptivity to the radiation therapy. You know that your body will work to kill and eliminate any cancer cells by allowing the radiation therapy to be very effective. As the radiation is absorbed into your body, all healthy cells will be protected by a special coating, while all cancer cells anywhere in your body will be hypersensitive to the radiation and will be killed off. Not a single cancer cell will survive. Your immune system is greatly enhanced and will help your body to eliminate and kill all cancer cells still present, if any, today and in the future, forever. Your love and acceptance of your own strength will allow you to mobilize your natural healing process to recover quickly. After the radiation therapy is complete, you will open your eyes and be wide awake, feeling relaxed and happy with an optimistic attitude because you know that the therapy was so successful. Time will pass quickly and pleasantly during your therapy. As each day goes by and you listen to this recording, your positive attitude will continue to enhance the healing process and the body's acceptance of the radiation.

Now you are achieving a peaceful, calm attitude, with no anger or fear of the future. You move instead to acceptance and the continuation of life. You may want to make changes in your life in the weeks or months ahead and this is wonderful, but for today you are only focused on being healed and happy and relaxed, fully accepting of the love of God, your family and others who say they love you deeply.

Each day as you listen to this recording, you reaccept the suggestions that are contained on the recording. They become more and more a part of you. Even though you may not consciously remember them, they will remain there in your subconscious mind and they will work better and more effectively than ever before. You will permit yourself to accept the suggestions in this exercise because you want to be cancer-free. You will allow yourself to accept the suggestions because you want to feel stronger, more in control, relaxed, healthier, and more vigorous. Your desire to be cancer-free, to be strong, and to take control of your life is so great that it easily allows you to accept the suggestions contained on this recording.

As you listen to this recording daily, you will feel more alert, refreshed, and relaxed, calm and refreshed, bright, sharp, physically better, emotionally better, mentally better and spiritually better than you have felt in a long time. These feelings of well-being will remain with you longer and longer with each time you listen to this recording. You truly feel more positive about yourself and the world in which you live. You look at things with a greater amount of faith that everything has a reason, and it will all work out in the end. You feel a higher force at work in your life, spiritually, which also facilitates the amount of faith you have. You make a difference in the areas you can, and release the rest. You feel more relaxed in each and every way. You feel wonderful now, self-empowered, more in control. Everything appears to work out more naturally during the course of life now. You're living more peacefully and naturally and are more relaxed than ever before.

Now take a moment and visualize, hear and feel yourself with a perfect cancer-free body, refreshed, bright, sharp, physically better, emotionally better, mentally better and spiritually better than you have felt in along time. These feelings of well-being will remain with you longer and longer with each time you listen to this recording. You truly feel more positive about yourself and the world in which you live. You look at things with a greater amount of faith that everything has a reason, and it will all work out in the end. You feel a higher force at work in your life, spiritually, which also facilitates the amount of faith you have. You make a difference in the areas you can, and release the rest. You feel more relaxed in each and every way. You feel wonderful now self-empowered, more in control. Everything appears to work out more naturally during the course of life now. You're living more peacefully and naturally and are more relaxed than ever before.

Now take a moment and visualize, hear and feel yourself with a perfect cancer free body.

Cancer Recovery: Tumor Reduction Imagery

Shark Eating Cancer Cells...

Now I want you to imagine there are sharks swimming in your bloodstream. These sharks are your friends. Notice that they represent your healing color. As they swim, they are searching for cancer cells, because this is what they eat. They feed on tumors and cancer cells. They've located where yours are in your body now, and they are starting to feed. You may feel a tingling sensation as they eat and chew...eating up the cancer cells in your body. They gnaw on all your tumors, several sharks at once, eating them up, gnawing, chewing, and continuing to devour them, Devouring them until they are all gone (pause). Now take the next few minutes to let this happen within your body...(long pause).

Melting Ice Cubes...

Now I want you to imagine that your tumors are like ice cubes. The spiritual light surrounding you is very healing and life-giving. It's also very warm. Now imagine that the light is penetrating the ice cubes, and as it does so, it begins to melt the outside of the ice cubes. The hot white light is now melting the ice cubes further as it shrinks them down. The outer layers of the tumors just drip away, and they get smaller, and smaller. Feel the ice cubes melting from the white light penetrating them. This higher loving light continues to melt the ice cubes down further and further as they continue to shrink (pause). Notice how this continues to happen as you just bask in the light (long pause).

White Light Meditation for Obtaining Spiritual Guidance

White Light Meditation

Separate your hands and feet and put your back into a comfortable position that it can stay in for a long period of time. Close your eyes and allow yourself to imagine a beautiful light emanating from the highest source in the universe...the brightest, highest, most pure light from the most beautiful and peaceful place. You know where this place is and can draw this light to you. You can feel yourself being drawn into the light as well. This light stands for everything that's good in life and beyond, such as unconditional love, peace, serenity, tranquility, and pure relaxation. Experiencing this wonderful light is your birthright, as you are from this place. Now you may safely unite with the vibrations of the light.

Allow this beautiful light to flow through every part of your being. As it flows through you from head to toe, allow it to completely relax every muscle. As it begins to flow through the forehead, feel that area simply relax. It automatically flows through the facial muscles and continues to flow down over the temples and through the front of the neck...at the same time down the back of the head, neck, and shoulders. Allow gravity to pull the shoulders down into their natural position. The mind may wander and drift, or it may become drowsy and foggy. Whatever happens is completely natural; you'll still hear the relaxing sound of my voice which is soon to become a comfortable feeling in the background. My words will soon blend together and flow into your mind naturally, so you'll be free from having to listen to the words because the subconscious will recognize what they mean anyway. Imagine that the mind is like a big whirlpool full of thoughts that have been swirling around, and now you can pull the plug and let those thoughts just drift and drain away.

Allow the white light to continue to flow through the arms and out the hands. The breathing becomes a shade deeper. With each more relaxing breath, feel the body resting with a safe, deeper, more peaceful sense of relaxation. As the white light flows down through the back, all the muscles and tendons wrapped around the vertebrae unwind and the back settles into its natural position. As it flows through the center of your being, notice that the light within you grows brighter and brighter. The part that has come from the light from within your center is now filling you and then emanating from you, as it intensifies. Feel your light surrounding you now with the light from the highest source. The light continues to flow through the waist, knees, ankles, and out through the toes. You and the light are one now...flowing within the same higher vibration.

Meditative Script

Now imagine that your mind can simply float up toward the bright light...floating higher and higher. And as you continue to allow your mind to travel up into the light, you may notice a number come to your mind. The number you hear, see, or feel is the number of spirit guides or angels that are there to assist you. Notice any other details about them...(pause). Now, completely blank your mind so that you may hear their message for you at this time. Just blank your mind now, and trust what comes...(long pause).

Child Birthing

New life is forming, growing, and moving within you. You are part of the promise and the destiny of life itself. A very important event is going to take place in your life, a normal, biological function. You're going to have a baby. What is happening now is a process of freeing the kicking, moving being who's been a part of your body for so long. Soon it will be time for the baby to become its own separate person. One cycle is ending and, immediately, another is beginning.

What has been called "labor" is the in-between condition, the fulcrum, the small time and space between two worlds. Change from one stage to another brings pressure, and then release. You will soon experience this also as the change is completed and fulfilled. You can feel this and embrace it and welcome it as refreshing and totally natural. With mind, you build a healthy attitude and happy expectation. Happy child-birthing has much to do with a healthy viewpoint. It is something remarkably beautiful. Being a channel of new life is said to be a holy experience. With this understanding and proper breathing, possible discomfort is lessened.

Later, as you begin labor, meditate on the tremendous universal force— the life force— you are participating with. Whenever you feel your body tightening up, actively think "release," "let go." There is a time for contraction and a time for letting go. Release, and welcome the process. You are learning to relax, flow, melt with the rhythm of life itself. With patience and positive expectation, all things are possible.

Happily picture yourself at an ocean beach. Watch the endless waves rushing to the shore— the ebb and flow of the sea. Observe it advancing and withdrawing over the sand. Become part of it; flowing into it, you become part of the rhythm of your own body, the tightening and releasing, the breathing in and breathing out, giving birth to your baby.

With appropriate physical and mental exercises, you are preparing yourself for this day of days. As you get into the rhythm and are working with your mind and body, the easier and smoother it becomes. Breathe as you've practiced in classes or read about. Each time you breathe in, breathe in "rest." Each time you breathe out, willfully breathe out any stress. Shift your focus away from the pressure to think of the final pleasure.

Mentally and emotionally feel yourself joyfully, totally aware, and participating. See it as already accomplished. Listen to that first sound of new life. Create a vivid symbol of bonding. (Pause)

You knew you could do it, and you did. You did well and it was wonderful. It is a healthy, beautiful child. Remember to savor each precious moment. Relax and flow with your body's natural rhythm.

After all, your body knows what it's doing. Just relax and let it do its job. Now observe in joy and amazement and watch the continuing mystery of creation unfold. The life force is now in you and with you.

(Complete your recording with the wake-up procedure.)

The Healing Bridge

In a moment, I want you to imagine two worlds, the one that you are in right now, and one that represents healing. You will need to exercise your imagination to be able to create these worlds within yourself as we do this meditation. The first world is the one that you have now. I want you to close your eyes and allow your mind to become light so that it rises up above your body now. Notice that your mind can float above the room and you can imagine everything down below through your mind's eye. As you float higher, you can float above the building, while still being able to see yourself and your room getting smaller and smaller down below. And as you float higher, into the clouds of the sky, you can locate anything and anyone on it from up there, higher, lighter, and floating. Now as you float above this earth, you are going to notice a translucent planet next to this one. In that world, everything is perfect and you are healed, and everything around you is just the way you want it.

There is a bridge that connects the two worlds that you can see. Float over the bridge now... You are going to land on the bridge on this side of the present earth for now. As you look at the bridge before you, notice what it is made of. Step onto the bridge and you will notice how it feels; you will hear voices or other sounds behind you, but there are even more interesting ones before you in the world of health and balance. It's very interesting over there, because you don't know for sure just how it will be there. It's more different over there than we would normally think it to be sometimes. So start walking across the bridge and you will notice a light beam at the end of the bridge, which you must walk through. When you walk through it, you will notice a feeling in the body and all the problems in the body simply disappear. The light has eliminated its problems. As you come out through the other side, you have a perfectly healthy body...a perfectly healthy body. Some things on this planet are very similar as before, but some have changed here in many ways; first you will walk down the street to your house... notice as you walk down the street what the neighborhood looks like.

You come across your house now. Notice how it looks on the outside. It's just perfect for you. It's perfect on the inside as well; everything is in harmony and balance as you walk up to the front door and step inside. You look around and you can tell that there is something synchronistic to why everything is just right. It feels great to be in this home. Everything is perfect there. Now you can sit down and relax in a favorite chair or go to a favorite room. There, you will notice that you feel a complete peace. You stay there for a little while because it feels like you have come home... you feel a tranquility and peace... Then you realize that it's time to go into another room of the house, which will transport you into a purpose; it may be a purpose you are familiar with, then again it may be a purpose that is completely different from the one you are familiar with. This purpose supports your home and loved ones, but it seems easy and perfect for you. It is something you simply enjoy doing. You really enjoy doing it, so as you step into that room you are really enjoying this thing that you do. You really like it. It's interesting, challenging, and you know that people simply enjoy it. On the planet of balance and healing, everybody you talk to respects and enjoys what you do, because it offers you and others value. You really like it there...

And now you are going to float above that world, into the sky above the home and purpose down below; higher and lighter as you float above that world you can see anything or anyone and everything and everyone is just fine there, as a very bright light from above continually shines upon everything. You will float back into the current world, taking the body, feelings, thoughts, and realizations back into the present moment. You are coming back with all of it and you will be spending a moment in each day understanding what it will take to bridge the two worlds. These ideas will pop into your mind and you will simply know what they are from a creative resource. When you come back into the present moment, you have a beautiful sense of well being. When you open your eyes within the next minute, you will feel wonderful.

Healing Imagery

As you relax further and further you'll begin to mentally shift your body with your imagination. You can create a metaphor now in your mind's eye that represents increased healing. You will be creative now and choose whatever comes to mind and focus on this image that represents increased healing for you. (Pause.)

Now brighten up the colors in the mind's eye and notice how much more clear the image appears... (Pause.)

Notice all the details you hear in the image and then turn up the volume so that you may experience these with more detail....(Pause.)

Now, imagine the feelings of increased healing. Notice the inward and outward feelings and sensations...(Pause.)

Now take some deep breaths. Inhale and hold a little while... and then exhale... Inhale again with a deep breath... and then exhale again. Repeat this several times until the sensation of stretching the chest and neck muscles begins to disappear, and these areas become naturally relaxed. Inhale... Exhale... Over and over, until deep breathing feels relaxing, refreshing, and very natural. As the chest cavity expands, you will notice that inhaling a large amount of air takes less and less effort. Notice how your posture improves from exercising your lungs. You sit straighter, you stand straighter. As you breathe deeper each day, your heart and lungs are healthier, working with less effort to send oxygen to every cell and tissue in the body. More oxygen going to the part of the body in need of rebuilding, restoring, and healing... remembering to breathe regularly and deeply, feeling more energetic, as you have more oxygen to your muscles, cells, and tissues with increased circulation, rapidly repairing.

This unique image is changing the body; it's training the body to respond to your thoughts now. You are overcoming any obstacles to healing with this image. You may notice that you think of this image often while you are in your room, your office, at your neighbor's home, your local shopping areas. You think of this image often because you want to have the healing occur more often. Your body wants you to do it. You give it that satisfaction, that natural satisfaction to your body now, because you deserve to improve it to the fullest level of health. Your body relaxes more deeply afterward. You feel more relaxed, less stressed; you forgot all about stress. You breathe out all your stress. Breathing deeply...relaxing. Breathing deeply and relaxing. You have more energy available. You are more aware of your body's needs and you are satisfying it more often, even if it's just minutes at a time.... You are allowing it to move more, breathe more, and heal more.

The body is responding, feeling better. You feel more balanced in mind, body, and spirit. You're taking care of your physical vehicle now and you have more value in your life. You're simply feeling good. You like your imagery adjustment technique. You like it, as changes seem to happen. You feel great!

Hypertension Recovery

Now one of the things you will teach your subconscious mind in the days ahead is how to relieve the causes and symptoms you have associated with high blood pressure. You know that there is a Christ centered core within your subconscious mind and body that is logical and rational, cool and collected, calm and relaxed, clever and wise, the one that wants you to heal and not have the hypertension or the symptoms of the hypertension or the underlying causes of the hypertension; this part of you is the part that wants you to be healed fully and completely. In, fact, it knows so much that even your conscious mind does not even know how much it knows. This Christ centered core has been there with you always and has helped you survive difficult predicaments in the past and will continue to help you in the future. This inner core that you know so well will help you heal the hypertension and the causes and symptoms of the hypertension. Now remember that from the beginning of time the subconscious mind and body have known how to heal themselves. The body knows how to heal over scrapes wounds and injuries, and how to generate new cells and new tissue when needed. The body knows how to regulate its own healthy functions such as heart rate and breathing. And with this knowledge, the body knows how to heal the high blood pressure and regulate the blood pressure to be normal. It also knows how to heal the causes in mind and body that may be causing the hypertension to manifest.

Now, In order to help to allow this inner healer and protector that you know so well, to maintain the optimal blood pressure for your body, you will develop an external signal for your subconscious mind. This will cause the body to make any adjustments quickly and immediately that will cause the blood pressure to return to normal levels. This external signal will go to your subconscious mind and cause the blood pressure to return to normal levels. This signal will be to put the thumb, index finger and middle finger of your left hand together, bow your head and take a deep breath. As you do this you will immediately become completely relaxed and you will feel the hypertension and the symptoms of the hypertension immediately leave your body. You will be joyous when this happens and you will know that each time you do this signal, it will become stronger and stronger until it becomes automatic. Over time you will be healed of all symptoms and all underlying causes of the hypertension. Your body will be whole, healthy and vigorous. You will feel very good about what you have and are accomplishing with the healing of your hypertension. You are thankful to the Christ within you that makes this healing and all healing possible. You are thankful to the universe for the gift of health, healing and love.

Over time as you continue to use your signal to become more and more relaxed and in balance with the world around you, you will let go of all stress, anxiety and fear associated with your condition. As you become more and more relaxed you will have the strength and confidence to reach the goal you have set for yourself to be free of any symptoms of the hypertension and the underlying causes of the symptoms today and in the future, forever. Your love and acceptance of your own strength will allow you to mobilize the natural, inner core healing process to be healed quickly and completely.

Now you know that this is a time for relaxation and healing. The more you allow your mind and body to relax, the more rapid and completely the healing will be. You can now allow yourself to permit your body to nurture itself and adjust and thus come into balance to enhance your body's natural healing process. Your desire to be healed and have a normal life enables you to gain the inner strength and energy within you to meet your goals. You have much to give and much to accomplish in your life.

Now as you listen to the relaxing sound of my voice, realize that you have the ability to release all cares, fears, worries or other negative thoughts associated with the hypertension. Right now all your cares, fears, worries and negative thinking will just drift away. In order to enhance the release of all negative thinking, imagine that you are near a large body of water. You may hear the water as it splashes against the shore. You may feel the coolness of a soft breeze off the water as it blows against your skin. You notice a boat nearby. Now I want you to put your thoughts and feelings of self-doubt, being scared, your excessive worry about the hypertension, feelings of helplessness, being overwhelmed and feelings of frustration on that boat; and allow it to drift off into the distance, off farther and farther away; so far and so distant that you can barely notice it. Allow it to be just a dot on the horizon. *However, you do not let the boat totally disappear because you may choose to retain these feelings and retrieve them if you need them. You can always bring the BOAT back. Right now, today, you have no need for these feelings.* As you let them go, you gain a sense of peace and calm flowing within your body.

You can now allow yourself the pleasure of watching those feelings drift further and further away into the horizon. *Notice that you do not allow them to entirely disappear, so that if you want those feelings back, they will be there.* Right now, you have no need for those feelings, so allow them to go off towards the horizon.

Now you are achieving a peaceful, calm attitude with no anger or fear of the future. You move instead to the acceptance of the continuation of life. Now, you may want to make changes in your life in the weeks or months ahead and this is wonderful, but for today you are only focused on being healed, happy, and relaxed, fully accepting of the love of God, your family and others that love you deeply.

Each day as you listen to this recording, you reaccept the suggestions that are included in this exercise. They are becoming more and more a part of you. You use your signal to become calm, peaceful and serene to remove all symptoms of hypertension from your body. Each time you use your signal you become better, better and better, more totally healed.

You will permit yourself to accept the suggestions in this exercise because you want to be free from the hypertension and all causes and symptoms of the hypertension. You want to feel stronger, more in control, relaxed, healthier and vigorous. Your desire to be completely healthy, to be strong, and to take control of your life is so great that it easily allows you to accept the suggestions and to use the signal that you have developed in this exercise.

Each time you do this exercise, you will feel more alert, refreshed, and relaxed, calm, bright, sharp, physically better, emotionally better, mentally better and spiritually better than you have felt in a long time. These feelings of well-being will remain with you longer and longer each time you do this exercise and each time you use your signal. You truly feel more positive about yourself and the world in which you live. You look at things with a greater amount of faith that everything has a reason, and that it will all work out in the end and you will be free of hypertension. You feel a higher force, the Christ force, at work in your life, which facilitates and supports the faith you have. You make a difference in the areas you can, and release the rest. You feel more relaxed in each and every way. You feel wonderful now, self-empowered, more in control. Everything is working out more naturally during the course of your life now and you are able to see yourself participating in all of the activities you enjoy. You're living more peacefully, naturally and are more relaxed than ever before. Now take a moment to feel and visualize yourself happy, content, at peace with life with a perfectly healthy body, free of all symptoms and causes of the symptoms of hypertension.

Preparing for Surgery

Sometimes I consciously hope and pray for the things I want in life, and sometimes I allow my subconscious mind to automatically accomplish things for me. As an example, I enjoy being alive. To live, I need oxygen; to get oxygen, I must breathe. I can pay attention to each breath consciously, if I so decide, or I can allow my subconscious to do this automatically.

In this relaxed state, I am discovering that there are many more things available than I have ever dreamed of. I feel a desire to allow my subconscious mind to help me at this important time of my life. I perceive that my subconscious may already be helping me without my conscious awareness, and what happens at a subconscious level is often more real, more automatic, and life-sustaining, if I simply allow it to help me.

No matter what any person believes, no matter what I consciously believe, the important thing is that my subconscious mind is working for me and for my successful operation. The subconscious mind can view reality through a different sense of time. I can, for example, review a happy scene from my childhood as if it were almost happening right now. It is easy to take a few moments and relive it. (Pause) I can also condense time or expand time.

I can also look ahead in time and, looking ahead, imagine that it has already happened. I can look at anything I wish and see it clearly. I can see myself having already gone into this surgery. My operation was successful in every way. My doctors and anesthesiologist automatically did the right things at the right time, and it all worked out fine.

Throughout the experience I was calm, peaceful, and confident. Some people afterward said that I was "cheerful." I slept comfortably and peacefully because I already knew how to calm my mind and put it on "automatic pilot." And even though I may have been unconscious, my subconscious mind responded to my body's needs and acted upon them correctly.

After the operation, the nurses made me feel safe, comfortable, and secure. I got plenty of rest and enjoyed the visits of family and friends. Total recovery was such a positive experience.

I am as a new person, refreshed, and heading for a healthy new future. Back home now with this very happy memory, I will look back next year and the year after that and say, "Thank God that it was all so easy."

I feel pleased in realizing that my subconscious did a great job, that I did a great job. Now it isn't really important for me to remember all that I accomplished here today; my subconscious mind understands it and, at the proper time, acts upon it. The information has been processed. I need not consciously know today that I experienced an "overview" of time and that I was perhaps completely anesthetized.

I realize that I am the author of my success. And soon, when I awaken, I may feel as if I were just waiting to begin.

Self-Health

See yourself floating in a vast, infinite, shoreless sea of glowing white light, an essence gentle as a morning mist. This is your own consciousness, your own mind, and you are learning to guide it, to make use of its healing energy. Feel this gentle healing light. Allow it to spread softly throughout your entire being. Bathe every muscle, every cell, every atom in soft, glowing healing energy. This healing light is alive within you and radiates from the deep recesses of your silent memory. Feel the warmth of this healing glow, its radiance—quiet, gentle, timeless. Feel it flow in gently spreading waves over every part of your body. Sense it growing brighter, stronger, warmer; bringing strength and vitality, excitement and happiness. Self-health is mainly a matter of mind. You are what you think you are. And you are now learning to restructure old attitudes. Strong, happy thoughts build a strong, happy body. Because good health is chiefly a state of mind, you can now consciously and subconsciously think healthy. Thinking healthy, you act healthy. Acting healthy, you become healthy. Illness prevention and sound health begin with attitude. You are what you eat, drink, and think. Choose carefully. A change of diet will not help you if you do not change your thoughts. Using the mind to consciously control the body is not a new idea. Eastern yogis, martial artists, and philosophers have been doing it for centuries. If you consciously control your thoughts and direct your mind in more tranquil directions, you can perceptibly influence heartbeat and blood pressure and reduce muscular tension. If worry, fear, anger, or depression strikes, the body reacts physically to what is essentially an emotional upset. Under stress, blood pressure soars, muscles tense and cramp, the stomach stirs, and the heart beats faster. All of this, of course, disrupts the body's equilibrium and weakens its resistance.

On the other hand, your body can now respond positively with a sense of peace and happiness. It can be relaxed, radiant, and alert. Medical science now recognizes that many common ailments originate in the mind, and often the most effective cure is the one that reconditions old attitudes. To perfect your body, start by perfecting your mind. To beautify your body, beautify your mind. As you program a healthy attitude, you realize that your body is the home of your mind and spirit. Your mind has the ability to repair its home as needed. Your mind and spirit are able to rejuvenate your body. The more you exercise your body, the more quickly it rejuvenates. Your attitude helps control how old you let your body grow. With sensible exercise, healthful diet, and a positive attitude, you can actually feel your body begin to feel younger. Rejuvenation is the act of becoming younger again. You have the ability to rejuvenate your body and heal the healer within yourself. Spirit, mind, and body are parts of the whole. An imbalance in one part creates blocks which affect other parts. Therefore, use your inner mind to create a spirit of health and to build a sound body. Your body is the servant of your inner mind.

Mind is the builder. Mind can build your body as your hands can build your home. Start with a strong foundation and design a comfortable appearance. Your body, like your home, can reflect your creative desire. Build carefully. Because every great achievement begins in the mind's imagination, you can use your imagination now to begin constructing a healthy new body. You have begun the process of rejuvenation and regeneration. If you form a mental image of yourself as you intend to be, you will feel healthy and happy and be filled with energy and stamina. Enjoy this picture of vibrant good health. Keep it foremost in your mind. *You are* healthy, energetic, and able to perform your physical activities. Hold this image or symbol of good health. (Pause) Imagine that it is already accomplished, and experience a feeling of feeling better. The information has been recorded.

Now tell your mind to make this vision reality. Tell your mind to make it happen; your mind can do it. What were once only wishes, you can now translate into reality. You are aware of this because you are doing it even now—keeping your mind happy and your body healthy. Healing happens on a physical, emotional, mental, or spiritual level—or it happens on all of these levels at the same time.

Surgery & Rapid Healing

Imagine where your higher power is, the very bright light that you feel exists above you. Imagine where this very pure, bright light is, and you will now release any fears you have into the light. The light will hold them or transform them there, but whatever it does, you trust and let go. Imagine locating any fears, tension, or worrying you've been storing within yourself and now release them into the light. You release them now, fully and completely. You will send a request to the light, your higher power now, asking that everything turn out the way it's supposed to... successfully; and you trust now that everything will be fine. You are going to do well. The medical staff is talented, well trained, well educated, and this is why they are there...so everything will turn out fine.

You are going to imagine everything will turn out fine. Everything will be successful for you and your body. Imagine that you are now being prepared for surgery, but you are relaxed, sometimes smiling, as you think of all of the positive benefits, you are in a good mood. You know your body will heal, heal rapidly, as you relax and let it do it's job. The healing forces will be stronger. Imagine you are going through the surgery for the next minute and everything is done just the way it was planned. (Pause) Afterward, you wake up with a positive attitude and the body is feeling fine. It is rapidly repairing, rebuilding, and relaxed. It is restoring its natural state of functioning more quickly now. You feel very relaxed and comfortable. You are relaxed and comfortable...letting the body restore its health on a cellular level; the tissue of the body--mending rapidly and healing over, so you are more comfortable with letting the body do its work naturally. You are comfortable. Any grogginess floats away rapidly, and your mind is more aware of everything in your environment. You may find that your mind is acutely aware of a favorite place that you are looking forward to visiting in the very near future. You feel fine in mind, body, and spirit now.

Wart Elimination

It is important for you to learn some things about yourself. You can learn that the flow of blood to the cells carries oxygen and nutrients to each cell, helping them to grow and multiply, to create new cells, to speed whatever healing must be done. And the most wonderful thing about this process is that you can learn to control it. This is something you can easily understand and begin to learn to do as you become aware of your physical body in a new and positive way. Healing can take place at any time. (Pause)

You can visualize the structure of a wart. You can see that it is useless and unnecessary. See the network of tiny veins and blood vessels that bring it nourishment. And now you can discover that, by closing off the veins and capillaries that feed it, you can deprive each wart of nourishment and nutrients. It receives no warmth, no attention, and begins to starve. And, in time, it shrinks; then vanishes, so that healthy new tissue can form in its place. Feel a sense of pride about yourself, your body, and the healing process. (Pause)

Take a deep breath now and think of healthy, pink new skin. As you let the breath out slowly, become aware of this new skin. Is it especially sensitive? Does it feel cool? Warm?

Beneath the skin are many veins and capillaries that carry blood and nourishment and warmth throughout your body—especially your (a localized area may be inserted; i.e., face, hands, feet, etc.). As you become aware of this, it is possible for you to actually feel the warmth, the blood vessels expanding to pump even more nourishment and oxygen through your skin. You can become aware of this and experience it in whatever way you wish. Perhaps you might recognize it as a pleasant tingling or a kind of soothing warmth. Now allow that warmth to fill you and experience new feelings in your body. You are learning a new awareness of yourself. You are discovering how to appreciate yourself, to accept yourself. And with this acceptance—the warmth and the attention—you feel more confident, more comfortable, more at ease, and pleased with yourself. Imagine yourself as you *can* look— not just one part, but your whole body. With a pleasant sense of awareness and a positive mental attitude, you experience warmth and healing energy.

Does the new skin feel tight or slightly tender? Notice the tissue underneath the skin. Can you feel the blood vessels pulsing as they carry nutrients to the cells? (Pause)

Imagine that you are resting on a secluded beach; really picture yourself at that beach under a bright sun shining on your entire body, especially on your (hand, feet, etc.) —a hot sun, getting hotter, with the heat penetrating your skin; a good feeling of heat that warms you completely with a soothing, penetrating warmth that brings healing; feeling warmth, with possibly a slight tenderness, as healthy new cells combine, pink skin forms, and the healing takes place. Now that your inner mind has recorded it, it is something you can experience at any time you wish. You can create this same feeling by simply slowing your breathing and visualizing the healing—thankful that it is already being accomplished.

Mountain Induction

Mountain Imagery...

I want you to imagine very clearly that you are relaxing next to a beautiful waterfall in a mountainous area. Perhaps you are supported by a rock or some soft peat moss — grass or what have you. Noticing the clouds drifting slowly across the sky. The sound of the water rushing over the rocks is very soothing. Perhaps there's a mist that feels cool and has a refreshing scent. The birds are singing as they bathe and drink within the puddles that fall upon the rocks at the sides of the waterfall. There's an awareness that it may taste like fresh-clear spring water. As the trees sway in the distance, you can hear the leaves clatter against one another creating one of nature's natural songs. As the sun rays of golden white light reflect off of the sparkling water, you can feel a pleasant warmth in the reflection upon your body. The sunlight stands for everything that's good and positive in life, such as love, peace, serenity, and tranquility—pure relaxation, growth, and prosperity.

Progressive relaxation...

Allow this light to flow through you relaxing every muscle fiber, cell and tissue. As it flows from head to toe, allow it to completely relax each muscle group. As it begins to flow through the forehead, feel the stress lines simply spread apart. It automatically continues to flow through the eyes as the thread muscles behind the eyes simply unravel and the eyes get heavier. The white light automatically continues to flow down over the temples and through the front of the neck...at the same time down the back of the head, neck and shoulders. Allow gravity to pull the shoulders down into their natural position. The mind may wander and drift, or it may become drowsy and foggy. Whatever happens is completely natural; you'll still hear the relaxing sound of my voice which is soon to become a comfortable feeling in the background. My words will soon blend into one another and flow into your mind naturally; so you'll be free from having to listen to the words as the subconscious will recognize what they mean anyway. And the mind simply unwinds like a big spring...letting go. As the sun rises on one side of the earth and sets on the other, each day is similar to one another with common themes. Each day has learning lessons of its own, regardless of the ups and down, moods, stresses...it has nothing to do with this. This is just pure-simple relaxation.

Allow the white light to continue to flow through the elbows, wrists, and out the fingers. You may notice a tingling sensation within the hands which further shows you're relaxing as the bodily functions are slowing down. The breathing becomes a shade deeper; with each more relaxing breath, feel the body rest more firmly against the pads that you're laying or sitting against. As the white light flows down through the back, all the muscles and tendons wrapped around the vertebrae unwind, and the back settles into its natural position automatically. The light flows through the waist, knees, ankles, and out through the toes, pushing out all stress, concerns, worries, in the form of tension or tightness, which may have been locked up in the body and are useless to us now. Feel the nerves dimming, like dimming the lights. And with each beat of the heart, that you're naturally more in touch with from becoming relaxed in this way, allow yourself to go deeper into relaxation. Feel all the muscles and tendons droop and hang on the bone structure, loose and limp.

Deepening techniques...

Therapy...

Awakening Procedures...

And now I'm going to count back from 5 to 1 and when I reach the number 1, you can then normalize.

> *Five*...You'll remember everything you have experienced.
> *Four*...Very satisfied with (the changes that have taken place).
> *Three*...More in touch with the room around you.
> *Two*...The mind and the body are returning back toward normal.
> When you imagine the number *One*...in your mind's eye within the next.
> minute, you'll become wide awake, refreshed, relaxed, and feeling good.

Ocean Induction

Ocean Imagery...

    Separate your hands and feet and put your back into a comfortable position that it can stay in for a long period of time. Close your eyes and allow yourself to imagine that you're approaching a beautiful beach on a bright sunny day, where the ocean seems like it goes on forever. Brighten up the color and notice how clear it is when you add all the details and how good it feels to be there. Feel the sand being the perfect temperature as it form-fits your feet. You may softly lie down in the sand or walk on the surf and listen to the waves as you watch them roll in toward you. There's a sailboat in the distance whose mast is teeter-tottering, back and forth. You hear the birds calling to one another, and the scent of the ocean mist is familiar in some way. The breeze is slightly cool, but the sun is nicely warm.

    A few clouds are drifting gently across the sky, a sky that goes on forever and the bright sunlight that reaches you shining down between the clouds allows you to feel warm and relaxed. This light stands for everything that's good in life, such as love, peace, serenity, tranquility, and pure relaxation.

Progressive Relaxation...

    Allow this light to flow through you, relaxing every muscle fiber, cell, and tissue. As it flows from head to toe, allow it to completely relax each muscle group. As it begins to flow through the forehead, feel the stress lines simply spread apart. It automatically continues to flow through the eyes as the thread muscles behind the eyes simply unravel and the eyes get heavier. The white light automatically continues to flow down over the temples and through the front of the neck...at the same time down the back of the head, neck, and shoulders. Allow gravity to pull the shoulders down into their natural position. The mind may wander and drift, or it may become drowsy and foggy. Whatever happens is completely natural; you'll still hear the relaxing sound of my voice which is soon to become a comfortable feeling in the background. My words will soon blend together and flow into your mind naturally, so you'll be free from having to listen to the words because the subconscious will recognize what they mean anyway. And the mind simply unwinds like a big spring...letting go. As the sun rises on one side of the earth and sets on the other, each day is similar to the next with common themes. Each day has learning lessons of its own, regardless of the ups and downs, moods, stresses...it has nothing to do with this. This is just pure, simple relaxation. All fears, guilts, and self-blame are released. Problems, pressures, and stresses built up through time are useless and unnecessary.

    Allow the white light to continue to flow through the elbows, wrists, and out the fingers. You may notice a tingling sensation in the hands, which further shows you're beginning to relax as the bodily functions are slowing down. The breathing becomes a shade deeper; with each more relaxing breath, feel the body rest more firmly against the pads that you're lying on or sitting against. As the white light flows down through the back, all the muscles and tendons wrapped around the vertebrae unwind, and the back settles into its natural position automatically. The light flows through the waist, knees, ankles, and out through the toes, pushing out all stress, concerns, worries, in the form of tension or tightness, which may have been locked up in the body and are useless to us now. Feel the nerves dimming, like dimming the lights. And with each beat of the heart, which you're naturally more in touch with from becoming relaxed in this way, allow yourself to go deeper into relaxation. Feel all the muscles and tendons droop and hang on the bone structure, loose and limp.

Deepening techniques...

Therapy...

Awakening Procedures...
And now I'm going to count back from 5 to 1 and when I reach the number 1, you can then normalize.
    Five...You'll remember everything you have experienced.
    Four...Very satisfied with the (changes that have taken place).
    Three...More in touch with the room around you.
    Two...The mind and the body are returning back toward normal.
    When you imagine the number *One*...in your mind's eye within the next minute,
    you'll become wide awake, refreshed, relaxed, and feeling good.

Safe Place Induction

Safe Place Imagery...

Separate your hands and feet and put your back into a comfortable position that it can stay in for a long period of time. Close your eyes and allow yourself to imagine a safe place in nature where you've been before or plan to be in the future; or you may just create it within yourself. Brighten up the color and notice how clear it is and how good it feels to be there. Notice the things that are moving about and how peaceful and wonderful the mood is. Hear the sounds of nature now, as they get a little louder. You may feel the warmth of the light in the sky, and the coolness of a gentle breeze. There may be a familiar scent in the air...a few clouds drifting gently across the sky, a sky that goes on forever, and a bright light that reaches you, shining down between the clouds...allowing you to feel warm and relaxed. This light stands for everything that's good in life, such as love, peace, serenity, tranquility, and pure relaxation.

Progressive Relaxation...

Allow this light to flow through you, relaxing every muscle fiber, cell, and tissue. As it flows through you from head to toe, allow it to completely relax each muscle group. As it begins to flow through the forehead, feel the stress lines simply spread apart. It automatically continues to flow through the eyes as the thread muscles behind the eyes simply unravel and the eyes get heavier. The white light automatically continues to flow down over the temples and through the front of the neck...at the same time down the back of the head, neck, and shoulders. Allow gravity to pull the shoulders down into their natural position. The mind may wander and drift or it may become drowsy and foggy. Whatever happens is completely natural; you'll still hear the relaxing sound of my voice, which is soon to become a comfortable feeling in the background. My words will soon blend together and flow into your mind naturally, so you'll be free from having to listen to the words because the subconscious will recognize what they mean anyway. And the mind simply unwinds like a big spring...letting go. As the sun rises on one side of the earth and sets on the other, each day is similar to the next with common themes. Each day has learning lessons of its own, regardless of the ups and downs, moods, stresses...it has nothing to do with this. This is just pure, simple relaxation. All fears, guilts, and self-blame are released. Problems, pressures, and stresses built up through time are useless and unnecessary.

Allow the white light to continue to flow through the elbows, wrists, and out the fingers. You may notice a tingling sensation in the hands, which further shows you're beginning to relax as the bodily functions are slowing down. The breathing becomes a shade deeper; with each more relaxing breath, feel the body rest more firmly against the pads that you're lying on or sitting against. As the white light flows down through the back, all the muscles and tendons wrapped around the vertebrae unwind, and the back settles into its natural position automatically. The light flows through the waist, knees, ankles, and out through the toes, pushing out all stress, concerns, worries, in the form of tension or tightness, which may have been locked up in the body and are useless to us now. Feel the nerves dimming, like dimming the lights. And with each beat of the heart, which you are naturally more in touch with as you become more relaxed in this way, allow yourself to go deeper into relaxation. Feel all the muscles and tendons droop and hang on the bone structure, loose and limp.

Deepening techniques...

Therapy...

Awakening Procedures...

And now I'm going to count back from 5 to 1 and when I reach the number 1, you can then normalize.

> *Five*...You'll remember everything you have experienced.
> *Four*...Very satisfied with the (changes that have taken place).
> *Three*...More in touch with the room around you.
> *Two*...The mind and the body are returning back toward normal.
> When you imagine the number *One*...in your mind's eye within the next
> minute, you'll become wide awake, refreshed, and feeling good.

White Light Induction

Imagery...

   Separate your hands and feet and put your back into a comfortable position that it can stay in for a long period of time. Close your eyes and allow yourself to imagine a beautiful light emanating from the highest source in the universe...the brightest, highest, most pure light from the most beautiful and peaceful place. You know where this place is and can draw this light to you. You can feel yourself being drawn into the light as well. This light stands for everything that's good in life and beyond, such as unconditional love, peace, serenity, tranquility, and pure relaxation. Experiencing this wonderful light is your birthright, as you are from this place. Now you may safely unite with the vibrations of the light.

Progressive relaxation...

   Allow this beautiful light to flow through every part of your being. As it flows through you from head to toe, allow it to completely relax every muscle. As it begins to flow through the forehead, feel that area simply relax. It automatically flows through the facial muscles and continues to flow down over the temples and through the front of the neck...at the same time down the back of the head, neck, and shoulders. Allow gravity to pull the shoulders down into their natural position. The mind may wander and drift or it may become drowsy and foggy. Whatever happens is completely natural; you'll still hear the relaxing sound of my voice, which is soon to become a comfortable feeling in the background. My words will soon blend together and flow into your mind naturally, so you'll be free from having to listen to the words because the subconscious will recognize what they mean anyway. Imagine that the mind is like a big whirlpool full of thoughts that have been swirling around, and now you can pull the plug and let those thoughts just drift and drain away.

   Allow the white light to continue to flow through the arms and out the hands. The breathing becomes a shade deeper. With each more relaxing breath, feel the body resting with a safe, deeper, more peaceful sense of relaxation. As the white light flows down through the back, all the muscles and tendons wrapped around the vertebrae unwind and the back settles into its natural position automatically. As it flows through the center of your being, notice that the light within you grows brighter and brighter. The part that has come from the light from within your center is now filling you and then emanating from you, as it intensifies. Feel your light surrounding you now with the light from the highest source. The light continues to flow through the waist, knees, ankles, and out through the toes. You and the light are one now...flowing within the same higher vibration.

Deepening techniques...

Therapy...

Awakening Procedures...
And now I'm going to count back from 5 to 1 and when I reach the number 1, you can then normalize.
   Five...You'll remember everything you have experienced.
   Four...Very satisfied with the (changes that have taken place).
   Three...More in touch with the room around you.
   Two...The mind and the body are returning back toward normal.
   When you imagine the number *One*...in your mind's eye within the next
   minute, you'll become wide awake, refreshed, and feeling good.

Chakra Induction

Separate your hands and feet and put your body into a comfortable position that it can stay in for a long period of time. Close your eyes and relax. I'd like you to imagine a rope emerging from your root chakra. The root chakra is at the base of your spine. This rope is going down through the carpeting, through the cement, and into the ground. It travels through the sand, the pebbles, the dirt, the stone, and down into the very center of the earth. When it reaches the center of the earth it hooks into a solid piece of rock and becomes very taunt. Almost like a steel pole.

Now I want you to imagine seeing a glowing white light. This white light comes to the base of the rope and attaches itself. It starts to travel up the rope - through the hard rock, through the stone, through the dirt, through the pebbles, through the sand, through the cement, through the carpeting, to your root chakra. This beautiful flowing light then starts to travel up through your body, filling you with it's serenity...through your sacral chakra, which is below your belly button, to your solar plexus...that place where you get that gut feeling and hold things in...to your heart chakra, and on to your throat chakra, then to your third eye...which is in the middle of your forehead, and up to your crown chakra. The crown chakra is a few inches above your head. When it reaches your crown chakra, the white light emerges like a fountain - this fountain totally surrounds you in this beautiful white light, protecting you from all forces and keeping you safe. Feel the feeling of warmth and security you find in this white fountain of light. Feel your body resting and going deeper into relaxation.

Deepening Techniques...

Therapy...

Awakening Procedures:

And now I'm going to count back from 5 to 1 and when I reach the number 1... you can then normalize.

Five ... You'll remember everything you have experienced.
Four .... Very satisfied with the (changes that have taken place).
Three .... More in touch with the room around you.
Two .... The mind and the body are returning back towards normal.
When you imagine the number One in your mind's eye within the next minute, you'll become wide awake, refreshed, and feeling good.

Alcohol Cessation

{Note: For the best results, therapeutic suggestions for the cessation of addiction to alcohol should be formulated from specific information that the client reports on the history of his/her addiction and life situation. Suggestions should also be formed from the diagnostic knowledge at the time of taking his/her nemesis, plus suggestions for building up his/her self-esteem and elevating his/her ego. After the induction of hypnosis, the following script, combined with suggestions specific to the client, may prove very useful in terminating alcoholism.}

(Induction...)

Feel relaxation growing and expanding inside you with each breath that you take and with each sound of my voice.

You may know that your mind is now peacefully and rapidly assuming the perfect level of relaxation to facilitate you becoming alcohol free, here today, forever!

First and foremost, I would like to congratulate you for deciding to walk away from alcohol. You have made this important, life-changing decision; you have decided to free yourself from the chains that have bound you to alcohol.

You may feel tremendous pride in the fact that you are forever walking away from this horrible, dangerous, and life-threatening habit. You are now walking away from the terrible control of alcohol on your work, your life, and your relationships. This is such an important day for you because you will now be reclaiming the best parts of yourself. It will be a marvelous awakening.

You are regaining your proper level of social prestige, and your correct place in society. Therefore, you can consider today even more important than your birthday. You may think of it as the day that you are being reborn. You can consider today the first day of the rest of your life!

To help you to fully understand how important this change is, and how necessary it is to your health and well-being, you may allow yourself to go through some important visualizations and mental processes along with me now.

First, you may now allow yourself to use your imagination.
Imagine that a color photograph has been taken of your liver.
Let's look at that sad picture together.
(Pause)

What do we really see? Well, I am going to explain it to you. As you can see, your poor liver appears to be badly enlarged and scarred because you have exposed it to the poisonous liquid, alcohol, day in, and day out, for years. Oh, your poor innocent liver! If only your liver could speak, what would it tell you? What would your liver have to say to you, if it could speak?

Second, I would like you to imagine that your liver has a voice of its own, and that it is actually speaking directly to you and saying, "Please look at me and see what has happened to me. For years you have made me the victim of your dangerous drinking habit by contaminating me with that poisonous liquid. Therefore, I have become sick, and as a result of that you have become vulnerable to all kinds of physical and mental problems.
Why don't you have mercy on me? Please show me some compassion. Please stop feeding me that poisonous, burning liquid, once and for all. Allow me to become rejuvenated. Let me heal. Allow me to regenerate and allow me to enable you to enjoy a good, healthy, and successful life."

Listen to your liver as it continues to speak to you and asks: "Have you ever considered the likelihood that

65

one day you will visit your doctor and your doctor will tell you that I have actually lost my ability to function? What will happen to you and me then? I'm so afraid of what you are doing to me, and to us! So, please stop feeding me that poisonous, burning, toxic liquid. Let me rejuvenate and I will help you enjoy a good healthy, happy, and successful life."

The question is, will you take this opportunity to respond positively to the sound of your innocent liver, by quitting this dirty, filthy, and dangerous habit?

Will you allow yourself the joy and pleasure of starting your life over again? Let your answer be "yes," and let the sound of that word, "yes," resonate in your mind, heart, and soul until it fills you with the certainty of your own ability to regain your health, your life, and a feeling of desire toward sobriety.

Right now you can consider yourself on the verge of a great psychological, physiological, and spiritual revolution. For this moment on, as you quit this dirty, filthy, dangerous habit for good, you feel completely reborn. Therefore, you can really consider today to be the first day of the rest of your life.

You can easily let go of this dirty, dangerous, demoralizing habit. You can emancipate yourself from the self-imposed slavery you've endured to alcohol.

You know that excessive use of alcohol can produce death in so many horrible ways, through gastritis, bleeding ulcers, pancreatitis, and frequently through cirrhosis.

You may now break free from the slavery, and free from the social stigma, and take your rightful place in society, and reclaim your health and happiness! You previously learned this dangerous habit through your unconscious mind, and today you are going to unlearn it in the same way you taught it to yourself. In other words, in the past, you inadvertently programmed your unconscious mind with this drinking habit, but today your unconscious mind will receive new messages that will enable you to become alcohol-free. Your unconscious mind is the seat of all your habits and the steering wheel of your behavior. Because your unconscious mind is now being approached through hypnotic relaxation with helpful and healing messages, you can and will unlearn this unwanted harmful habit and feel reborn today.

Did you know that alcohol will weaken your libido, robbing you of your sexual potency, decreasing your sexual performance, and perhaps even destroying your sexual desire?

Alcohol causes your brain cells to die and leads to lapse of memory, amnesia, and loss of intellect, and perhaps even loss of life.

Isn't it time to walk away from this filthy, dangerous, enslaving habit? Isn't it time to stop ingesting that poisonous liquid which renders you out of control, damages your social prestige, and ruins your life?

So, please, let it go! Release it now! Start enjoying a good, healthy, happy, and successful life. There is no reason to remain a slave to such a dangerous habit. Take a moment to consider a very important point in this change. Is there anybody in the world who likes to be controlled by another person? The answer, of course, is "No!" You wouldn't allow yourself to be controlled by another person for a single hour. But, even though you wouldn't allow another person to control you for even an hour, you have allowed that poisonous liquid, alcohol, to control you for years.

Thankfully, that is all over now. From this day forward, you will be free of the addiction, free of the social stigma and feelings of despair, free of the nagging hangovers, and lapses of memory. Free!

You deserve to be congratulated. You can feel confident that the whole ordeal has now come to an end. You may allow yourself to forget that alcohol was ever a priority in your life! Take another moment to consider that from the very first moment you began to drink that poisonous liquid, you became a loser. Due to this dangerous habit, you have crippled your social standing, robbed yourself of energy, and weakened your self-esteem.

You have worked hard to earn your money, and then you have wasted it on this poison. It has been like you have been setting fire to your own body. But now you deserve to be congratulated. From the moment you stop this dirty, filthy habit, you are a winner! By eliminating this dangerous habit, you regain your health, your energy,

66

and your productivity.

You have wasted your hard earned money by setting fire to your body with this poisonous liquid long enough. Congratulations, you have made up your mind just at the right time, before this dangerously poisonous habit could cause any permanent damage to your physical or mental health. You are making this important change in time to prevent further damage to yourself, your family, and your social status.

You are feeling better about yourself because you decided to stop this harmful habit. Therefore, from now on, day by day you will feel better and better. From now on, you will take care of your health and feel an overall sense of well-being. Congratulations! From this moment on, you are a liberated person, and you can really start to enjoy the beauty of life.

In fact, let's take a moment to envision your wonderful new alcohol-free life. Picture yourself getting up in the morning—with a clear head, and hangover free. Notice how motivated and productive you feel. See yourself moving happily through life free of alcohol. See yourself engaging in new healthy activities. See yourself getting through a wide variety of activities - and feeling happy to be free of alcohol. That's right, you are able to easily function in any and all situations - free of alcohol.

Your sense of purpose and your levels of health and happiness have dramatically increased since you became alcohol-free. Your liver and brain cells are functioning better each day now that you are alcohol-free. Your confidence and self-esteem grow each day and you continually feel better about yourself, your relationships with others, and your place in the world.

Allow your mind to experience and enjoy what your life will be like as you become alcohol-free. Fill in the details of how you want to look and feel, and of what your life will be like when you are alcohol-free. Feel yourself stepping into that picture and know that in just a few brief moments it will become your reality.
(Pause)
From now on, whenever you see someone drinking, you will hate its sight, smell, and taste so much that it will be difficult for you to imagine that there had been a time in the past when you have been dependent on this poison.

Yes, from now on, any form of this ugly liquid will be so distasteful and disgusting to you that you will be reluctant to even imagine using it, or even touching it, ever again. The thought of alcohol is so totally disgusting to you that you will forever be glad to be free of it. From this moment forward, whenever you do anything that was previously done while drinking alcohol, you will be reminded of the reasons that you kicked the habit, and you will be able to enjoy that activity without alcohol. You will be reminded of all the problems alcohol caused you and you will enjoy the experience of being a nondrinker.

You will enjoy the feeling of being sober and alcohol free, so much more. Feel totally confident that there is no force in this world that could cause you to touch this poisonous liquid ever again. The drinking problem has now gone down in your history as one of the unwanted detrimental habits of your life that you overcame.

Now, you realize deep inside yourself that you have completely dropped this dangerous habit. From now on, whenever the thought of drinking crosses your mind, you instantly relax, relax, relax, and feel good about the fact that you are alcohol-free.

You actually feel proud of yourself for eliminating such a dangerous habit. You feel good that you have walked away from the social stigma. You may now concentrate all the energy you formerly wasted on alcohol addiction into constructive arenas which boost your ego, enhance your self-esteem, and raise your spirits. You feel totally confident that this dirty, unwanted past problem has been left far, far behind, and that every muscle, every fiber, every nerve, and every tendon in your body has become counterconditioned to this dangerously poisonous habit.

Allergy Release

As you continue to relax, notice how your mind and your body are already beginning to relax. You feel more comfortable as your body loosens, and relaxes. And now I want you to take a few deep breaths, as you do, each deep breath fills your nasal passages with comfort, with contentment, your nose, lips, mouth and nasal passages relax automatically more with each breath. As you breathe out, you breathe away all tension and tightness. Just easing it out and away from your body.

As you breathe in, you're allowing all doubt to fade away. As you breath in now, take the feeling of relaxations deep into your body, into your lungs, as it passes into your blood stream, where it is distributed to every cell in your body, allowing health and healing to move into every cell of your body. As that vital life force passes through your body, begin thinking about the parts of your body that used to overreact to allergens in the past; and as you think about the parts, you relax more deeply, more completely in each of those areas.

And now imagine the word "allergy." Medically, the word "allergy" or "allergic" pertains to a condition or sensitivity to some substance. A person who is allergic overreacts to substances. Allergic reactions are actually a normal protective action of the body, however, there are times when it is being misused by the body. Now we are going to let that misuse go. We are going to release the body from overreacting. You will now relax around any foreign substances, take them into or on the body, and then cease reacting. You're going to cease reacting. You will relax as you touch it, take it in, simply release any overreaction. You will react normally now. Every cell in your body will accept the substances that you used to be allergic to. It will accept these substances as normal and unobtrusive. It will take them in as normal and unobtrusive. Relaxing with them and releasing them normally, with a normal reaction of cleansing them from your system without infection, cleansing easily and normally. Relaxing and letting go.

As you let these substances leave your mind and body now, you will come to realize that anything that the mind causes, the mind can also cure. Your subconscious mind is understanding this fact as all of your body's processes will now function properly, cleansing all impurities out of your body and eliminating the allergy symptoms you have been experiencing and no longer need. You are going to notice a change in your life, because your mind is releasing those thoughts, ideas, imprints and impressions that caused the allergies to develop in the first place. You are releasing any past reasons, any past need for the allergies. Your usual pattern of being allergic will never be the same again. Beginning right now, your subconscious mind is understanding that you want to get rid of all unnatural overreaction to allergies. Your subconscious mind is understanding that the information received about allergies was misunderstood and you want it understood correctly now, from a more knowledgeable, more mature, point of view, and you want it changed and corrected. You want the process of your body to function properly and cleanse all impurities and substances which have any allergic element out of your body through natural, normal processes through your elimination system. Your subconscious mind is causing you to become desensitized to all substances and situations which in the past have caused you to suffer allergic reactions. You refuse to have those unnatural reactions, and your subconscious mind is getting rid of the habit of responding that way.

You'll continue to relax your lungs and sinuses even more now as your subconscious mind is accepting my suggestions and is improving your health enabling you to live your life in a more peaceful, calm, more relaxed way. Each day these suggestions become more effective. You're learning to use these principles of relaxation which you are now experiencing in all phases of your daily life, and that will keep you calm and relaxed at all times. In every situation or circumstance that comes up where you used to be allergic, instead, you will be calm, relaxed, your nerves will be relaxed and steady, and you will be able to function in a relaxed way, putting the past beliefs of overreacting out of your mind. You will be able to cope with your everyday changing circumstances, in a loving, peaceful way. Regardless of what comes up in your life, you will be in more control of your emotions and feelings, and that will cause your immune system to be void of overreacting, and all allergic responses will soon be gone completely.

And now as you take a deep breath easily and effortlessly, filling your lungs and sinuses with fresh air and relaxation, you begin the healing and repair process now. Your heart is strong; it is beating strong and regular, bathing every cell in your immune system with the awareness of normal responses. You are comfortable and serene as you feel the air going deeply now sending oxygen to bathe every cell with peace and tranquility. Every organ, every body system is functioning perfectly well on its own now. As your body and your mind work perfectly together like a finely tuned instrument, creating health, peace, a calmness and tranquility, you feel your favorite music go through your lungs and sinuses. You are confident, calm, serene, and relaxed, your mind and body are relaxed with under-responding to substances from the past. Now your brain and mind are giving perfect directions to your body; healing and restoring itself to normal, calm, and healthy responses to the things around you now and in the future.

Now you are in control of your body's responses. You can control the systems of your body. You have a new sense of being, and a new sense of wellness within. Now you are going to imagine being exposed to a substance you used to overreact to, but you are going to relax with it, allowing the substance to be present while your body adapts to a wellness condition, taking it in, stabilizing, and then releasing it through normal body systems...cleansing, healing, and letting go.

Anxiety

...and now that you are learning to relax, you will begin to find ways to stop anxiety and relax more often. You will teach your mind to stop anxious thoughts and focus...focus on more productive and positive thoughts. You will notice in the days ahead that you are exercising control over your subconscious thoughts. From time to time when repetitive questioning...questioning yourself, your world, situations, and your mind is racing, you will tell it to "stop!" You will tell it to stop because you want control over this. You are going to become a little more assertive with your subconscious mind by telling it to "stop that!" You are going to say, "Stop!" if you have to. You are going to notice that your subconscious mind is going to listen to you now. You have control. When you say, "stop" it stops. When you say, "don't do that," it listens. It stops, it quiets itself, and then you slip in a true and positive future oriented message. When it stops, and you give yourself a break, you then give yourself a true and positive oriented message, then your mind focuses on the future, the future the way you would like it to occur. When you get the positive future message, you stop there. When the future image or message feels right to you, you stop there, focus, breathe deeply and slowly and you move on to something you'd rather do or think about. You've reached at least a temporary resolution now, and you stop there. You've thought about it long enough, and now you relax the body, with deeply relaxed, slow breaths and you find that there are other more relaxing and positive ideas you'd rather focus on.

You gave it enough time, now you will simply change the channel of the mind, like changing the channel on a TV set, moving forward to something more interesting and relaxing that you can focus on. Once the channel of the mind changes, you are done with your previous thoughts and you move on, you move on to the next thing. If any mind racing, or anxiety in the body happens again at any time in the future, you will forcefully tell it to stop, quit that channel and change the frequency of the mind to something else, and the body will respond. The body will respond with natural-easy relaxation. You have other things you'd rather do or think about in the future. Your focus is more positive now. You only allow a very short period of time for anxious thinking, reach at least a temporary resolution and move on with your thoughts, move on with your life...

Because of this ability, you have a new lease on life. Positive messages about yourself and your world will enter into your mind more frequently during your waking hours. Even in your dreams, there will be more positive outcomes. You will sleep better, dream better. You will release the things that you can't immediately change. You will move your focus away from the things you have no control over, and instead, focus on the things that you do have control over. You now have control over your mind, your anxiety. You can stop it and focus on more productive things. You have a higher self image, and higher self esteem. You truly feel more positive about yourself and the world in which you live. You look at things with a greater amount of faith that everything has a reason, and it will all work out in the end. You feel a higher force at work in your life, spiritually, which also facilitates the amount of faith you have. The higher forces will take care of things, and you begin to notice how things unfold on their own this way sometimes. You notice small ways in which the higher forces intervene in certain places and situations in this world, and so you release control over worldly cares to the higher forces. You make a difference in the areas you can, and you release the rest. You feel more relaxed each and every day this way. You feel wonderful now. Self empowered, more self control. Everything seems to work out more naturally during the course of life now. You're living more peacefully and naturally. You're relaxed now, more often, a much more relaxed person.

Attracting Abundance

What is abundance to me? As I evaluate material success, I realize that abundance is a good thing and that I am worthy of it. I perceive that I am entitled to life's many blessings. But to me abundance is much more than merely money or things; abundance is in having good friends and in being a good friend. Abundance is a harmonious life, a music-filled home, creative work, a meaningful relationship, quiet inner peace with strength and spiritual growth. I will enter into a new age, and for me this new age is the age of abundance.

I see abundance all around me. In nature—in the fields and the forests, the rivers, the seas, deep within the earth and high in the sky—there is abundance for all.

I feel abundance in and around me. It is here and it is now. I welcome this abundance with joy and delight.

In my creative imagination I see an economic healing happening. It seems a miracle! I have been blessed with abundance. I have opened an inner door and stepped into the sunlight of abundance in all its manifestations. And I say "thank you" for this great gift. For I know that it comes, not from me, but through me. And with this new abundance, I can grow and serve that I may be a channel of blessings to others, for abundance is an expression of love.

I have tuned in to the aura of abundance that surrounds me. Like the electromagnetic field of a magnet which extends beyond the magnet itself, so it is with my energy field, reaching out far beyond the actual physical me. And, as a magnet, it draws abundance to me. It attracts and guides me to abundance. And this I now do:

To attract abundance I now act and think as one who already has abundance. I smile often and easily. I enjoy taking time for the little things and the quiet things in life. I walk tall and proud and perhaps just a little faster now. I have many exciting new habits reflecting this abundance.

To attract abundance I take good care of my physical appearance. But I take even better care to balance my inner appearance. I am aware now to choose my spoken words carefully, but I am even more considerate of my unspoken words. I use positive, cheerful words easily and often, for they reflect the profound, positive, cheerful feelings deep inside of me.

To attract abundance, I praise others for the good that they do. I compliment others honestly and sincerely. I thank others lavishly. I compliment and thank myself also, and welcome this new me. I like listening attentively to others, and they enjoy listening to me.

To attract abundance, I find meaning and joy in the work that I do, my activities, and my service to others. Work is love in action, so I happily do more and contribute more than I am paid for. My creative work is a pleasure and a fulfillment. But, if my present job is void of creativity and promise, then I can analyze the alternatives and take the steps necessary for a rewarding new career in whatever field I choose.

To attract abundance, I carefully make lists of my goals, my ideals, and my plans—especially my plan of action. I write out in detail what I will accomplish, how I will accomplish it, and when I will accomplish it. I make realistic short-range goals and I make reasonable long-range goals, and then I simply go out and do it, and I often believe that I am far ahead of my goals.

71

To attract abundance, I make friends and associate with positive, creative, and active people; for I realize that I am always influenced by the people around me and with me. So it is vital that I choose wisely those with whom I work and play, live, love and grow. Positive, happy people encourage me and inspire me as I encourage and inspire them.

To attract abundance, I clean out all excess clutter in my life. I phase out all trash. I give away my neglected things that others may use them. I make room for the many, many blessings coming my way. I joyfully bestow my blessings by sharing my excess abundance with others. And, as the useless and the unwanted depart, I experience the freedom and the lightness of an unburdened life. What then comes in to fill the void spaces will be a joy and a delight.

To attract abundance, I allow myself to laugh often and to laugh loudly. My sense of humor has expanded into a habit of laughter. With happiness and laughter, I attract new friends, positive people who laugh and enjoy life with me. With joy and laughter, I improve my health and appearance. I laugh and the world laughs with me. I make people laugh each and every day, for laughter is like an internal massage.

To attract abundance, I open my doors wide when opportunities knock and I welcome them with open arms. My life now is exciting and active, and many, many blessings come to my door. If nothing succeeds like success, then nothing is more abundant than abundance.

I open the door to the joyful discussion of abundance.

I open the door to my actions and thoughts of abundance.

I open the door to my caring for my outer and inner appearance.

I open the door to praising others and myself.

I open the door to new joy in my creative work.

I open the door to listing my goals, ideals, and my plans for action.

I open the door to expanding my world of friends.

I open the door to releasing the excesses in my life.

I open the door to joy and laughter.

I open the door to the new me—today—now, and it is so!

In my creative imagination I can see a clear, sharp image of myself attracting abundance. I take time to review my ideals and goals. (Pause) I hear friends congratulating me on my successes. (Pause) I feel a total enrichment has already been accomplished.

Now I realize the great secret of abundance: Abundance is not an end in itself, but a growing process, the result of my creative work and efforts. I have learned from the past, make plans for the future but live in the eternal now. I already have abundance and, by the joyous welcoming and sharing of abundance with others, I increase my abundance a hundredfold.

Career Planning

You can be anything you want to be. But you don't have to be anything you don't want to be. You can consciously choose to do anything you want to do. Or, in due time, your subconscious may guide you to endeavors that utilize your natural inner abilities. At this level you begin to discover innate talents and inner knowledge that can be applied to any area of your life.

Some people need ample time to realize their inner gifts. Other people have so many natural talents that they need time to decide which ones they wish to pursue actively. Some people hurry in pursuit of a career, when often they need but to be still, to listen first, and be open to life's opportunities. By carefully choosing to slow down your outer mind, you gain new awareness and guidance in your *inner mind*. Some people write out a list of things they plan to do, and a list of things they wish not to do. Like a patient fisherman, some people cast out their lines in many directions to see from which places responses come. The wise fisherman knows that though there may be no response one day, the very same spot may be alive the next day. Life is like fishing; with persistence and patience, all things are accomplished. What you are doing now in your spare time gives insight into what you will be doing later on. Time, even spare time, is an energy to be used wisely. As you breathe in and quiet your thoughts, new insight, new directions form deep within you, symbols of your new self. It doesn't matter if this is perceptible to you right now or not. All that is important right now is that you have a deep desire to apply yourself in a brave new way, that you want to step out of old ruts and worn patterns. As you dare to believe, as you trust in life, as you listen to your subconscious, you realize that your future is determined by the careful and wise choices you make now.

In your creative imagination, look ahead and see yourself near the autumn of your life. You are older and far wiser now, more experienced, and can review your entire life from this perspective. As you mentally look back upon your life, ask yourself, "In what way do I wish to be remembered?" "Have I served and helped others?" "Have I been honest in my dealings?" Especially ask, "How have I used my life?" and "Am I pleased with myself?" Your higher self truly knows the best directions. You can follow its lead and act upon your inner feelings. Your inner self becomes your best authority. Soon you will really understand what the best directions in life are for you. Follow them.

Confidence for Success

You have come to a point in your life where you are preparing to move beyond any fear or blockages to your ability to have success. You are tired of getting close and not following through; so now you are going to make a promise to yourself to focus on fully succeeding and allowing yourself to experience the joyous feeling of being a successful person. You will have an innate ability to approach any goal or situation from this day forward, and be able to move through it. You are looking forward to completing yourself within it. The suggestion to be successful will go deep into your unconscious mind now. Relax... breathe deeply and easily, and now you will train your mind and body to relax and focus on the idea of success. Train your mind to think of a time when you were successful at something. You think now only about this success where you were happy. As you imagine this, you realize that you deserved to be successful. You can notice some colors there that were present when you were successful in the past. You can imagine some sounds that remind you of success. You can imagine a feeling of success in your body. The environment is just right for success. You are totally relaxed now, as you imagine your past success. Notice how you can see, hear, or feel your past success. You feel very natural there.

Now, find this feeling of success in your body. This beautiful and natural place of success and accomplishment is within you; you can locate this memory within your self and it makes you relax... relax naturally and automatically. Whenever you think of this success memory, you relax automatically. Notice that you know where this memory is in your body and you are going to move this peaceful memory to the location in the body where you used to feel your fear. You move it to the place where you used to feel the fear. The fear feeling in the body disperses now. It is replace with this very successful feeling, the knowledge of what it is like to be successful. The success grows within you. You have a right to be successful. You have a right to complete things all the way. You think about it, you locate it in your body, and you're there. You feel success. Whenever you think about your success memory, you will relax. Regardless of where you are, you will experience confidence automatically. Your mind will re-member success, relaxation, contentment, and you will have confidence that you can and will succeed at the right moment, when the opportunity presents itself. You will also find yourself unconsciously and automatically creating opportunities to succeed.

Now imagine that you are in the future. You are experiencing an opportunity to succeed and you would have normally felt anxious about it, but instead, you feel relaxed and confident as you follow through to experience the success you deserve. You remember that you've succeeded before. You are relaxed and more confident with the idea of success. You are confident in the future situation where you used to feel fear, but instead you are relaxed, confident with a higher level of concentration. You are relaxed and you feel great because you are accomplishing your goals of following through to be success-ful. Imagine how wonderful you feel as you simply relax with a higher level of confidence in your abilities, having a focused concentration level. You feel capable. You feel self assured, confident, relaxed, and successful. You know that everything is going to be OK this time. You feel an exhilaration from succeeding at this with little concern, or practically fear-free, as you relax and create ways to move through any blocks to success. Imagine now that you have been successful. Afterward, you have a wonderful feeling of success, self accomplishment, greater self-confidence and a wonderful sense of freedom.

You feel great even now, because just thinking about it now, you know you are more relaxed with the whole idea. You are at peace and in control. Your fear has disappeared. You let it go. You are relaxed now. You are relaxed, confident, at peace with the idea. You're at peace with this... peacefully, relaxed.

Developing a Sense of Humor

At times I have taken myself and my world too seriously. And at other times I burst forth with laughter and joy. How special are the times when I simply let go and roar a hearty laugh. What great release and expression! Sometimes I have laughed so much that my sides seemed to split, and this causes more laughter, and I just let my body laugh even more when this happens.

I feel better after a good laugh. Laughter is good for my body— it is like an internal massage. Today I express a little lightness, a bit of levity, a smile, a cheerful word, a hope, a song of joy— and this becomes a pleasurable habit, a positive way of life.

Sometimes I am most comical when I take myself too seriously. Humor balances the extremes of my life and puts things in proper perspective. When ego becomes punctured or puffed, if I plop to a depressing low, I'll just smile and laugh—and let it all go. Humor is my saving grace that helps me to laugh at myself and see my all-too-human folly.

My eyes and my mouth express my humor, and my face radiates with joy— but my face merely reflects what is already within my mind and heart. Humor and joy begin within and express outward. I look for the funny, the silly, and even the ridiculous.

A smile is said to be one of life's greatest assets. It can work miracles by transforming me, by relieving tensions, strengthening bonds and brightening my outlook. I am forming a positive habit of smiling often and smiling with delight. Smiling costs little and pays well. Smiling expresses humor, grows into laughter, blossoms into joy. Joy is my expression of appreciation and thankfulness. My joy is alive with profound creative force.

In my creative imagination I am picturing how positively the world responds to my smile and my warm humor. I am visualizing how good I look and feel when I smile and laugh. My laughter is a positive symbol of my happiness. . . joy is an emblem of my life; laughter builds love, and humor affirms my humanity. The picture of this already accomplished is very clear.

Ending a Relationship

Shakespeare said, "All the world's a stage, and all the men and women merely players. They have their exits and their entrances. . ." Sometimes people visit our lives and, while they are here, we can welcome them and enjoy their company and carry happy memories of them when it's time for them to go—even when it seems there may be some disappointment attached to it. You are beginning to learn that life is like a drama.

By turns, the curtain rises to open an act— the curtain comes down to close an act— but the play goes on, with new actors and new excitement, and all kinds of wonderful experiences to enjoy, places to go, people to meet and different things to do.

I wonder if you can imagine a curtain being raised and everything is changed. Now the set is different, a new scene is beginning— with possibly a pleasant sense of excitement and anticipation—as you discover all the things that are waiting for you. Perhaps you can pretend you've just come to the earth, and life begins with your next breath, and everything is fresh and alive. (Pause)

You know how to remember certain people, certain experiences, even though at times it seems you can forget them.

You know how to remember. Now you can begin to discover that, in due time, you will think of [him/her] less often, but always with pleasant recollections of happy times you shared— blessing the passage of this relationship and all that you have learned from it.

Very soon now, something new is going to happen. You will meet someone, and day by day [he/she] will take up more of your thoughts. Sometimes you may even try to think of your past relationship and discover that your thoughts go to this someone new and special, someone who is even nicer, who brings you happier feelings, whom you are truly more deserving of. And you will learn again just how exciting a new discovery can be.

The old act has ended. And, by turns, the curtain rises again, for you have earned the right to experience and enjoy a better relationship. Imagine your life all fresh and new. You live each day fully, learning from the past without regretting it, as you enjoy today; looking forward to your tomorrows with happy expectation.

The curtain opens; you take your place and the action begins. In fact, it has *already* begun.

Enhancing Creativity

If you take a deep breath and exhale it very slowly, you can visualize your breath like the ocean with the waves coming and going. And, as the waves ebb and flow, so does your breath come in and go out. Allow yourself to rest upon the shore, and imagine all the weight leaving your physical body. Imagine yourself beginning to float safely, bit by bit. Allow yourself to float comfortably a little bit more above where you are resting. Enjoy this wonderful feeling of rising up and pleasantly floating on the air.

As you are enjoying this feeling of floating, you become more aware of your inner self. You can visit parts of your inner self and look into the deep recesses of your mind. You can look on things from your past and gain knowledge and learn—positively. Allow yourself to sense and feel rather than merely think. Your heart and your emotions are doors to your creativity. Allow your inner knowledge—your stored memories—and hidden talents to unfold through your feelings and emotions, for through the avenue of the heart you gain new insight and inspiration.

Begin to feel the quiet radiance of light and life surrounding you. Let yourself hear the harmony that is you becoming in tune with creation, with the spirit within. Be still and listen to this inner voice; it tells you of new awareness and new perceptions.

Your inner voice encourages you to enter your special Creativity Room. You hear your inner voice saying: "This is my ideal space for growth and development. I come here for inspiration and insight. This is my inner place to be intimate with my creativity. I have access to a wealth of information and talents. I detach myself and redefine my perceptions."

In this Creativity Room your inner mind creates mental images, clear pictures of creative insight. The right image will come to you. Create a symbol of your success. These creative insights can also come in on their own—any time, day or night. Symbols come through dreams or sudden flashes; and, because they can be subtle and fleeting, you can have pen and paper ready to write them down. Exploring the dream state, you better understand the symbolism and simplicity of your inner wisdom.

Your nighttime dreams and your daydreams can bring new inspiration and expression beyond your present understanding. Look within to these creative insights, visions, and illuminations to discover more fullness of life. Picture yourself and feel yourself using this creative process. Spell out your objectives, and then wait and listen to the voice and symbols of the inner self. Allow creative mind to give you the answer. Answers can come quickly or slowly.

The more you use this creative process, the quicker and easier it all becomes. You will think beyond your present way of thinking and act beyond your present mode of action. You are already using more of your creative potential—it is already happening. Utilize this creativity and bring it back with you, as a symbol, a stream of consciousness, or a new way to do things.

You can slowly return from your venture upward. Returning, settling gently and softly back on the beach, watching the waves and the sea.

Finding Lost Objects Cycle

Before looking back on time and events, you can allow yourself to become completely relaxed. In your creative imagination mentally visualize the misplaced item, and see yourself as having already found it— perhaps right where you originally set it, or where someone else subsequently moved it. All that is important now is that you "feel" and reunite yourself mentally with the article.

Literally feel it back in your hands and avoid thinking about just "how," but just do it. Simply feel it; sense it as if it is already here. (Pause) Take your time.

As a detached observer, you may start going back through time to before the article was misplaced. You'll discover that it is easy and pleasant to do this.

Reliving is always interesting— a pleasant, enjoyable exercise. Slowly look around and sense the place and time; this is your time to retrace your actions. At this deep level of relaxation, this higher level of awareness, it is easy for you to reexperience.

Take your time; take all the time you want, and slowly review the chain of events as you see them, as you feel them. Realize that some people see a memory, others hear a memory, and still others feel or sense a memory.

All that is important now is that it is interesting for you to recall or relive events of the day, step by step, or in slow motion, as you follow along, understanding what you did, how you did it, and why. As you tune in to the events, using your mind as a mental zoom lens, focusing in on the exact scene and activity, the more vivid it all becomes, seeing pertinent actions and clear pictures.

In a little while—when you awaken, as you get up— in due time you can go and recover the item. Much to your amazement, the object will not be in the first place you search, but you can discover it at the second place you look. You will be pleased with your success and thankful for the return of your goods.

Infertility

You are surrounded by a divine blue healing light, which is flowing through all of your body. You have the power and ability to control your body. Your body is filled with positive energy. Your mind is all-powerful and you now use it to help with the conception of your baby. Conception is brought into existence when the sperm from the male fuses with the egg from the female. Picture this in your mind's eye... your ovary is releasing a perfect egg, which travels smoothly down the fallopian tube. This egg fuses with the sperm from the male successfully. A single cell is then formed. This single cell then undergoes the first of many cell divisions until it forms a cluster, which will eventually implant itself in the lining of the womb and mark the start of pregnancy.

Again, picture this in your mind's eye...your body has released a perfect egg. It is successfully united with the sperm from a male. It then forms a single cell that forms a cluster and then implants itself in the lining of the womb and your child is now growing perfectly within your womb. You will have a successful pregnancy. You will feel perfect. Your child will grow perfectly within you. You will become pregnant. Everything is perfect. See everything inside of you as perfect and your perfect baby is forming.

Feel how happy you are. See and feel your baby as it grows inside of you, knowing with a warm glow of confidence that you have been specially chosen for this honor.

You will, in a few minutes awaken with the full knowledge that you will become pregnant and you are at peace with yourself.

Memory/Comprehension Script

And now that you're more relaxed, your subconscious will remember how easy it is to become pleasantly relaxed just by thinking about familiar-relaxing ideas. You are capable of using your innate ability to relax in any situation. You will relax and remember naturally when you want to. When it comes to (tests or performing), you will remember by listening to your subconscious and simply recognizing the things that you are familiar with. Just by relaxing, you will become more clear minded, and it will feel more natural to let ideas flow into your mind, trusting your thoughts, trusting *yourself* more than ever before.

Your mind is like a camera; it takes pictures through your eyes. You're becoming more visual as you store the pictures taken with your eyes in the subconscious mind. Everything you've seen before, therefore, you will recall just by recognizing the pictures brought to you in the form of memory. As you relax and let your subconscious bring you the pictures at the right time, the most correct answers will appear to you automatically, more easily, and with more confidence. You'll recognize the picture that pops into your mind and simply trust the answer.

Your mind is like a recording as it records everything through the ears. You're becoming more auditory as you store the sounds that your ears have sent to the subconscious mind. Everything you've heard before is recorded in the subconscious mind...very similar to a tape or CD recorder. Everything you've heard before will be available to you as your subconscious replays all the important messages. It's easy to simply relax and allow your subconscious mind to play the tape or CD back to you as you listen for the answer. Therefore, you will hear and recognize the correct answers automatically, more easily, and with more confidence.

Your mind is also full of impulses. You're becoming more aware of the way you feel about specific subject matters as the subconscious responds to them. When topics are brought to your attention, your subconscious records the feelings associated with them and you trust the feelings within your memory. When the subject matter appears to you again, you will recognize the positive feeling or learning and choose the most correct answer automatically, more easily, and with confidence.

Now remember, any past experiences involving your unpleasant memory experiences are insignificant, so let bygones be bygones. So notice how you forget to even think about those things, releasing them now... releasing. Unpleasant performance memories disappear as quickly as a breath of fresh air.

A nice deep breath completely relaxes and focuses you anywhere at anytime. Breathing... relaxing... and focusing your attention automatically. Your concentration level will be like a laser beam cutting through metal. You're focused. You're relaxed. You're confident.

Take a moment now to remember a time when your memory worked very well for you. You remembered something important; yes, you did it successfully before in another situation.... When it comes to (tests or performances), you'll succeed as you've also succeeded before in other areas of your life. You've succeeded in other situations that you put your energy into. You made things work before because you have the ability to succeed. In the very near future, you will be able to relax and enjoy being attentive to your memory functions, automatically, more easily, and with more confidence. Listening to the pictures, tapes or CDs, or feelings within the subconscious may even seem to be a game of fun and challenge. Studying is simply letting the subconscious absorb the information and testing is simply relaxing and being aware of the subconscious process of retrieval. And because you're willing to relax and listen to yourself, you will trust yourself more than ever before, feel more self confident, self assured.

You're going to be much more relaxed and more successful than ever before. You have a lot to look forward to...now imagine yourself after the (test or performance) when it's all over and you feel very relaxed, confident, satisfied and at peace with yourself. You may be saying to yourself, "I did it. I knew I could do it."... and now there's a wonderful feeling of success and self accomplishment.

Overachievers

Take a deep breath and breathe out. Feel yourself relaxing. Hear the words "calm" and "relaxed" echoing through your being. You are calm and relaxed, you are feeling wonderful. Imagine, now, soothing bath water slowly covering you— gentle warmth enveloping you— first, your feet, then your legs, your stomach, your chest, neck and head. You are calm and totally at peace.

You are breathing easily and naturally as ever; all cares are absorbed into the water, and you are totally limp. Every muscle is soothed by the subtle rhythm of the water as it lulls and caresses every inch of you. You're floating, lighter than you've ever felt before, allowing the water to take you here and there with its gentle flowing motion— in and out again, soft, rolling, soothing, quieting your mind, separating you from all pressure and responsibilities, cradling you in peace and harmony, in a place that is totally filled with tranquility. Flow with the gentle lapping of waves on a sandy shore, being a part of that action, a part of the water, feeling rhythm of constant harmonious ins and outs. Now, with a count of one to ten, you will become even more relaxed and at ease...one. . .two. . .three. . .four. . .five. . .six. . .seven. . .eight. . . nine. . .ten.

You are a goal-oriented person. You have many plans and projects to improve your work and your life. You are a high-energy person and you love life. You take pleasure in living life to its fullest each day; and, because of this natural, exuberant energy that you have, there are times when you may have forgotten to allow your body to rest fully. Life is filled with ups and downs, a balance of summer and winter, of rain and sunshine. You need both the highs and the lows in order to understand this balance. You may have become preoccupied with one aspect and neglected the other. This is easy enough to understand. Perhaps you have been driving yourself too hard in order to achieve a specific goal. But now you realize that balance is in order, because intense driving and pushing actually delivers a reverse effect. Built-up kinetic energy feeds on itself, until it can spurt energy in random directions. But this was in the past. Now you simplify your life.

You are understanding your energy patterns now and are able to harness, control, and release your life's energy in exactly the way you want to. Look at yourself closely. Note the instances when you experienced this state of overabundant energy. You can realize that this oscillating energy was at times wasted and counterproductive to your needs and goals. Whenever this feeling comes, take a moment to close your eyes and count from one to ten Feel the tension releasing, and feel your body relaxing into its normal equilibrium, your maximum productive state of calmness and poise. Give yourself, allow yourself, this moment of diversion, this relief from all efforts and mental pressures. Simply feel relaxed, and now it will be easier than ever to organize and synthesize your plans and activities, because you've renewed yourself and given your body needed rest from physical or mental work.

Now it will be easier than ever to handle your responsibilities more effectively than before, because you can be whatever you want to be. You can calm yourself and relax your mind and body whenever the need arises. You can also set time aside each day, each week, for the enjoyment of your many successes, and make time to appreciate your blessings. Even after this session is over, each time you count from one to ten, with practice you can enter this same state of calm relaxation that you are experiencing right now. Recognize and rejoice that you have such abundance of energy at your disposal and realize that it is easy to harmonize this energy and balance it in such a way that it allows you to attain maximum benefit.

Picture yourself as the calm, relaxed person you wish to be. Experience this as already having been accomplished and know deeply that you *can* be anything you wish to be. You can be calm, relaxed, poised, and in control of your energy in every situation.

Preparing for Change

I feel a need for change—in my body, in my mind, in my soul, and in my emotions. I am ready to accept life's continuing process of change, forming a new pattern to learn and grow, welcoming change in all levels of my life.

As I prepare for this continuing process of change, I will remember and analyze past changes and observe that each change was a lesson to be learned and was necessary for my growth. As I continue to study past changes, I will realize that often what were the most challenging changes were, in truth, the *greatest opportunities* for my personal growth.

And, in dealing with human emotions, I realize that in the past I may have felt I was the victim of change. But now I am the instigator of change. Now, rather than meekly waiting for change, I can and will initiate change. I can make it happen. I will fill my changing with a positive and realistic attitude and accept that each change brings with it levels of growing that are necessary and good for me to experience.

I understand the need for constant change and self betterment. I can visualize this as a home which has not been cleaned, repaired or remodeled, but has been left to deteriorate. Or, as I would look upon a neighborhood which has not progressed, but has fallen apart. Or even a city or a nation which refuses to change and becomes stagnant. This process of change is ongoing, up and down, through generations of peoples, eras, and seasons. Sometimes there seems to be no "middle ground," no safe place to avoid change. This is especially true with me, so I will plan on progress, I will welcome change, and I will build my future.

Change must come into each life, as day must follow night. What I *do now* determines what my changes will be and how I can grow with them. I bring my goals and ideals together into one vivid symbol or picture of how I will grow and become stronger and more loving. The right image will come and I will focus on this clear picture.

The greater and more profound the changes, the greater and more dynamic is my strength to meet these changes and grow through them. I release and set free the burden of negative emotions, whether self inflicted or not, which I have felt from persons or events in my past. I release the feelings which I have imposed upon myself and held. As I forgive and bless other people—and release these emotions—I feel better and more positive about myself. I am confident in the future I am planting seeds. The seeds of my tomorrow are in my thoughts, my plans, my words, my touch, and my actions.

I wholeheartedly embrace the joyous responsibility of change in my life by liking myself, by taking care of my body, by letting my emotions grow constructively and by lovingly sharing my joy with others. In the eternal *now I* am becoming a more positive person. I bless those who have taken care of me in the past and those who will share my life in the future. I give and receive blessings each day and grow to be a happier, more loving person with each season of change in my life. And, I bless myself for caring about myself and my growth. I develop my will to change and my will to succeed. I have created a new habit of joyfully welcoming change at all levels of my life. I appreciate change, for it brings new opportunities for positive action.

I am thankful for the many positive changes which have already happened within me, around me, and through me. I am thankful for the exciting changes yet to come. I welcome them, knowing that the continuity of life is change. I am becoming all that I am capable of being.

Public Speaking

I can be anything I want to be. I can really understand how to feel good talking to other people. I am becoming an effective speaker.

Emotion is a good thing; it is an element of being human. I enjoy that element, but emotion is not enjoyable if it prevents me from expressing myself openly in a clear, logical way. If there had been times in the past when, through emotional stress, I may have been unable to communicate easily, I realize this *was* all in the past.

Now that I am becoming an effective speaker, I understand that the inner feelings which I may have experienced are simply adrenaline— my body's own abundant, natural energy, available for my use, available for me to harness and control at the right time, to accomplish any goal I set for myself.

Controlled adrenaline can keep me sharp and aware; I can direct and channel it into enthusiasm and vitality. I can become whatever I want to become, and, with this realization, I am becoming a successful public speaker. I allow my own innate sensing mechanism to let me do the right thing at the right time, to let me say the right thing at the right time.

I speak clearly, precisely, calmly, and effectively in a way that people can enjoy and easily relate to. In my mind I can visualize myself standing in front of an audience, preparing to speak. I take a deep breath and feel myself continuing to breathe easily. Smiling, I take a moment to look at the group of people.

My thoughts are coming into focus, they are distinct and well organized, because I am cognizant of what I am going to say to get my point across.

I am an effective speaker; I am sure of myself because I have prepared my material and am familiar with it. I see myself as calm and vividly focus on this positive assured image in my mind. (Pause)

I am an experienced speaker, expressing myself delightfully in every situation. This is an enjoyable and exciting experience because I concentrate on what I am giving to the group. I clearly deliver each important point to my audience. I am simple, yet direct. As I am speaking to the people, I am loving them and serving them— giving my gifts— aware of what I am sharing, helping them to learn and grow. Expressing the full and profound magnetism of my soul. I feel this as having already been accomplished. I am thanking the audience for this opportunity to share and be with them. (Pause)

I now picture myself *after* the talk. Smiling people are coming up and thanking me, saying how much they enjoyed and learned from the talk. As they are shaking my hand, I realize that I truly did well. I did do a good job and am thankful for the experience of helping others and speaking with them.

(Complete your tape or CD with the wake-up procedure.)

Self Esteem/Image Classroom

...You're walking down a long hallway now and come upon a door. The door is marked, classroom of the mind. You open the door, eager to look inside of the subconscious depths of your mind from where all your negative messages and impulses come from. As you walk through the door, you notice a chalk board with all of the negative messages that have been given to you in the past. These labels and messages have slowed you down; and they have failed to reflect the good, worthy, and valuable person that you truly are today. You can begin now to erase these messages one at a time. Erase these messages now one label at a time, one sentence at a time, from any age, from any time, from any person... Erase them all so that these all turn to chalk dust, one at a time, all chalk dust (pause).

Now, the only thing left of these in the depth of the mind is a blank black board, a blank black board where they used to be. Now I want you to begin to write positive messages that truly reflect your abilities and your personality characteristics. In this space you begin to write words that describe your positive attributes. You can pick from a wide variety of attributes that may include things like, intelligent, talented, creative, sincere, honest, valuable, confident, helpful, skilled, capable, and even more that cross your mind now (pause).

Image now, that there is a TV set in another part of the room that is showing you future successful scenes from important areas of your life. You can just have a seat and watch the future successes as they begin to play on the TV screen now, where your self esteem and self image is much higher, much higher. The first scene is where you are standing tall and proud of yourself as you are a good friend to another person. You are a good and valuable friend and you are confident in the things you have to say. You are speaking your truth and you feel confident that what you are saying is valuable. You are a good person with good intentions for people who are your friends. You feel yourself being a good, worthwhile person and are sharing this feeling with others more easily now.

Imagine yourself talking now to coworkers, bosses or employees. You know you have special talents and ideas to share that are valuable for yourself and others; so you're able to express these things with more confidence, more confidence in your abilities, self assured, and speaking your truth more freely. You're more confident with your talents and abilities. You have more appeal as you speak with greater comfort. You are more comfortable with sharing your abilities and contributions with others. Your conversations are easier now and people are respecting what you have to say more. They value the things you say. People are regarding you as a valuable and respectable person. They want to hear what you have to say. They are interested in your ideas. Imagine that you are more assertive, more self assured, more confident in sharing your ideas, and people want to hear you. People want to see you as you hold your self differently. Your voice is more relaxed in your chest. You breathe easier as you speak. Your posture is straight and tall. You hold your head high, and you like who you are. You like who you are and so others naturally like you too. You have appeal and you are kind to yourself now. You say nice things to yourself on a regular basis. You don't have any time for negative thoughts and feelings anymore. You put those out of your mind. You fill your mind with positive messages now. You feel more positive with positive thoughts, you look more positive, you sound more positive. You like who you are now with positive reminders of yourself flooding your mind more often. You have a positive self image and you are kind to yourself now as a very worthwhile person. You feel fine. You feel just fine now with a new positive self image.

You are going to leave the TV set behind you in the class room of the mind now, and as you leave the room you will notice that the door behind you stays open. You are leaving the deeper levels of the subconscious mind open to these positive messages and experiences so that they come to you more often now during a normal day. The door is left open for a lot of new positive messages and feelings that will come to you often...

Self-Sabotage Script

Recognize the difference in what you "actually" do and in what you feel you "should" do. Live up to responsibilities and face up to the responsibilities that you owe to yourself.

Instead of repeating behaviors that fail to help you, you do what helps you. Self-deprecation is useless. Putting yourself down is totally unnecessary and putting up road-blocks to success is absolutely and totally unneeded.

There are solutions to your problems. Look for answers within yourself. Start to overturn negative pictures or thoughts. You DO have workable tools to change your thinking and to change your life!

Repeatedly remind yourself — "I have created my world and I have created my thoughts, so I can change by selecting how I perceive and react to my world." Perceptions and reactions are a choice.

You can increase and enhance the talents you already have to help you. You are able to develop new skills to manifest good things in your life. Explore the actions and choices you are making so that you can develop perspective and attain encouragement to solve difficulties. If you are your own stumbling block, then one-by-one, block-by-block, remove the obstacles.

Look at and examine on all levels your choices, decisions, and motives without judgment and without criticism. In the immediate future, you gradually develop more and more confidence in yourself and in your abilities. You CAN alter undesirable habits, traits, and attitudes. By improving or positively changing your way of thinking, you can change your life.

Emotional handicaps can and will be overcome. You are totally capable of making a conscious decision to overturn self-defeating thoughts or activities. Eliminate old negative influences and negative beliefs from your mind. You are a worthwhile person. Allow yourself self-satisfaction. You do have the ability, skills, and talents to eliminate negative habits or negative tendencies.

Self-defeating patterns can and will be broken because you are worthy of what is good and beneficial for you. Give yourself the permission to succeed and enjoy success.

Sleep Well

I want you to imagine a whirlpool that is swirling around in your mind. In this whirlpool are thoughts of the past of yesterday, or yesteryear. These are the thoughts that no longer serve you and that keep swirling around, circling, swirling... These thoughts may include stresses from living the natural course of life. These are things that may not change, may take a long time to change, or require resolution; and these are thoughts you are going to learn to release so that you can give your body the rest that it deserves. They may also include unpleasant experiences of the past, guilt, blame, shame, fears, or whatever crosses the mind. Because these are all unnecessary and unnatural messages and experiences that have been standing in your way of your natural God-given right to sleep, I want you to pull the plug now. Pull the plug and let all of these thoughts from the past just drift and drain away. Let them all get sucked down the drain now as you pull the plug, swirling down and drift and drain away. Every last negative thought just drifts and drains away (pause).

As you relax more deeply now, deeper and deeper, you will make a promise to yourself that will help you sleep... This promise is that you will only think of resolving stress during your alert time. Your alert time is when you want to be awake, when you really need to be awake. You agree to think about resolutions and problem solving only during your alert time. So for now, you release all stresses, concerns, and so on... you release them to a higher light, imagine a higher light, a spiritual light. This light is likely to be where you have come from and to where you will return to... It's your right to be connected to the light. As you focus on it, it gets brighter and brighter. You feel its warmth and peace. You allow its warmth and peace to reach your body now. It feels relaxing, serene, peaceful, and very tranquil. You allow this light to relax your body, and you release all tensions that may have been trapped in your body to the light. You release all your tensions into the light where it will hold them, and be given the chance to transform them. You release all your cares from your mind now into the light. In the light these thoughts may be given the chance to be suspended there for now, or perhaps transformed there. You let them all go, for now. Out of the mind; out of the body.

Released from your spirit, you let them go. The light wants you to do this, so you let them go. And as you release all tensions in the form of thoughts and feelings, you relax more deeply, much more deeply. Your breathing reaches a new relaxed level or deep, deep sleepiness. Your mind begins to drift as you allow it to sleep, sleep; you may even say the word "sleep" to yourself, as your mind drifts, drifts deeper. The mind drifts and wanders into a deep direction, of deep sleep and the body relaxes to a deep, deeper level now. The body just starts to melt into the pads that you're laying against. Your body simply lets go, simply lets go. You relax, sleep, as your body gets heavier and allows the pads to support all of your weight now. The pads want to support your body, and your body simply starts to float into a new direction of deep, deep sleep. You are sleeping more deeply now. You are falling asleep more quickly in the future and you release and let go. You are staying asleep longer now, because if you should happen to awaken, briefly, you tell yourself that you are simply going back to sleep, and to your body, this is natural. Your mind will give the message to your body to go back to sleep, so that you sleep all the way through until you need to get up. You tell your body that it's OK now to sleep, sleep all the way through until it needs to come back from sleep land. You will feel well rested at that time, well rested. You exercise your natural God-given right to sleep. Your inherent spiritual ability given to you at birth to sleep like a baby. To sleep naturally.

So your body will want to get more rest, more often in the future. You have more confidence now that you can just let your mind and body do what's natural, more often. You simply trust that your mind and body will do what's natural to let go, release yourself fully and completely to sleep, natural sleep...simply letting go. Trusting that you can simply let go now. Fully and naturally sleeping. You feel better during your waking hours; and you can think more clearly because you now have the ability to sleep, sleep naturally.

Classroom of the Mind

Imagine that you are walking down a school hallway in an effort to educate your mind for success. You come upon a doorway marked, "Classroom of the mind." As you open the door you'll notice two chalk boards, one to the right of you and one to the left of you. You notice that the one to the right has a bunch of words on it. These words are negative statements that you have been telling yourself, false statements that fall far short of your abilities.

But now that you've located these subconscious messages, you can erase them. Take the opportunity now to pick up an eraser and erase all of the negative messages. (Pause) Now they have all disappeared into chalk dust and out of the mind.

Then you walk to the chalk board on the left and pick up a piece of chalk and begin to write one positive message after another. These positive messages are things that you need to tell yourself that are true about your abilities... positive messages. They are all very positive, as you write one after another. Some of them may be future abilities now... just write them in now, all of them. (Pause.)

Now you are going to notice a video projector in the back of the room with a large screen. When I say the number one, you will press play on the projector and notice that you are the star performer on the video. You are going to be watching yourself perform everything that you've wanted to perform perfectly now. Every move on the video is perfect. You are relaxed and focused watching yourself be relaxed and focused in the video. When I say the number 10, the video will be at the end. One, two, three, four, five, six, seven, eight, nine, ten. Now hit rewind and then it's quickly back to the beginning. Now hit play and watch yourself again. One, two, three, four, five, six, seven, eight, nine, ten. Now press rewind and you're back to the beginning.

This time when you see the video, you are going to jump into it and experience everything around in full color, with full sound and feelings of success. Press play now... One, two, three, four, five, six, seven, eight, nine, ten. Very good. You have trained your mind how to help you become a success. Everything went perfectly. You will be relaxed and focused in the future when you perform everything successfully. Your concentration will be like a laser-beam cutting through metal. You will be focused, relaxed, and successful.

Stress Relief-1

One of the things you will train your subconscious mind to do, in the days ahead, is how to release stress. Stress comes from the conscious mind focusing itself on stress rehearsal. Stress rehearsal is a stressful situation from the past, or one you may encounter in the future. It's a natural process so that you may reach resolution, but unnecessary stress comes from too much stress rehearsal. When too much stress rehearsal occurs, you may start to drain your energy, worry, encounter self doubt, and so on. You are going to stop this overuse of stress rehearsal by making a promise to yourself. You will only give a stressful thought a short period of time. This time period may be one or two minutes, or maybe even up to 15 minutes sometimes, but you will never exceed the time period you promise yourself. You will only think of stresses for a very short period of time, reaching at least a temporary resolution, and then you think of something else you'd rather do or think about. You begin to say to yourself, "That's enough." You find the positive learning lesson from the stressful thought, give yourself some credit for finding value in it, and you focus on something positive. You focus on something else that makes you feel good about yourself, your life. You begin to notice that you close down negative thinking earlier, and you begin to focus on positive thinking. You use your think time more wisely with positive outcome thinking.

You gave negative stressful thinking enough time, now you will simply change the channel of the mind, like changing the channel on a TV set, moving forward to something more interesting and relaxing that you can focus on. Once the channel of the mind changes, you are done with your previous thoughts and you move on, you move on to the next thing. If any mind racing, or anxiety in the body happens again at any time in the future, you will forcefully tell it to stop, quit that channel and change the frequency of the mind to something else, and the body will respond. The body will respond with natural-easy relaxation. You have other things you'd rather do or think about in the future. Your focus is more positive now. You only allow a very short period of time for anxious thinking, reach at least a temporary resolution and move on with your thoughts, move on with your life...

Because of this ability, you have a new lease on life. Positive messages about yourself and your world will enter into your mind more frequently during your waking hours. Even in your dreams, there will be more positive outcomes. You will sleep better, dream better. You will release the things that you can't immediately change. You will move your focus away from the things you have no control over, and instead, focus on the things that you do have control over. You now have control over your mind, your anxiety. You can stop it and focus on more productive things. You have a higher self image, and higher self esteem. You truly feel more positive about yourself and the world in which you live. You look at things with a greater amount of faith that everything has a reason, and it will all work out in the end. You feel a higher force at work in your life, spiritually, which also facilitates the amount of faith you have. You make a difference in the areas you can, and you release the rest. You feel more relaxed each and every day this way. You feel wonderful now. Self empowered, more self control. Everything seems to work out more naturally during the course of life now. You're living more peacefully and naturally. You're relaxed now, more often, a much more relaxed person.

Stress Relief-2

You begin to release stresses now that you have no control over. You will notice that you are changing your life-style to release the stresses of which you have no control. You begin to notice areas of your life that are stressors, but that you have control over. You have control over the decision as to whether or not you will expose yourself to certain stressful people or situations. You begin to notice that you are imagining certain people that stress you on a TV screen. You are looking at them from a distance... and you are noticing that there are times when you can make a choice to spend less time in their immediate presence. Notice each person on the TV screen from your most comfortable chair in your TV room that you can simply imagine positive future outcomes for each person which would have been stressful for you, but you changed it by avoiding them, or resolving their influence on you. Notice, as I pause for two minutes, you are about to find ways to do this with each person that crosses your mind. (Pause)

Now notice that you are able to watch stressful situations on your TV, and within the next moment, you will find ways to avoid those situations, or resolve those situations. Take two minutes to notice positive future outcomes for each situation which would have been stressful, but you changed it by avoiding it, or resolving it. (Pause)

And now if you noticed that some people or situations had not had an immediate resolution in you mind, you will release them. You will begin to release them to a higher power. Imagine a very bright, pure and warm light now. Imagine where the higher power, God-force exists. Because you come from this light, I want you to bring it closer to you. You may feel yourself getting closer to it now. You have a right to connect with this higher light now as you meditate on it. Keep focusing on it, and the warmth and peace of this light will get stronger. (pause)

Now I want you to locate the place within yourself where you've been holding those people and situations that you cannot change. Find those within you now, and I want you to continue to focus on the brightness of the light, because you are going to release them into the light. The light will take them and either hold them or take them to transform them in its own unique way. You can release them into the light and feel much better now. You are going to disconnect any attachments, ties, or threads or cords that connect you to these things, by imagining you are cutting these ties, cutting these ties safely with a big pair of scissors and releasing them completely and fully into the light. As they drift up higher and higher, they drift away from you now. They drift far away and into the light. You feel better now, much better.

You look at things with a greater amount of faith that everything has a reason, and it will all work out in the end. You feel a higher force at work in your life, spiritually, which also facilitates the amount of faith you have. The higher forces will take care of things, and you begin to notice how things unfold on their own this way sometimes. You notice small ways in which the higher forces intervened in certain places and situations in this world, and so you release control over worldly cares to the higher forces. You make a difference in the areas you can, and you release the rest. You feel more relaxed each and every day this way.

Stress Management

As I realize that I am now deeply relaxed, I can also achieve this relaxation at other times and places. When I take a few minutes and close my eyes, I can reexperience this calm feeling whenever I wish. And, as I practice this daily, this calmness, this harmony, becomes a part of my life.

When I close my eyes for a few minutes and, stepping back, take a deep breath, I can mentally say and repeat the word "relax." I then achieve internal centering or quieting. This simple exercise helps balance my actions with my thoughts and my thoughts with my actions. And then, the more demands that are put on me, the more strength I have when I open my eyes and, stepping forward, meet the situation.

Through these moments of quiet that I am practicing, I am understanding myself and others better. I learn to rise above stressful situations by working toward the best solution and not being held down by the problem or by my real or imagined fears of it. I am learning to keep my ideals and goals always in sight by focusing on the greater good to be achieved beyond the obstacles.

I am experiencing harmony on a physical level, a mental level, an emotional level, and a spiritual level. As I step toward peace and fulfillment on each level, I become a happier, healthier, more loving person— stronger within myself—and, therefore, more able to cope with the world.

As a mental exercise, I can imagine myself as an automobile. I can start my day, as I start my car; then, slowly and carefully, I shift into higher gear. I am aware of the traffic and the conditions around me. I take the best roads toward my daily objective and make careful choices at new intersections. Most of the time, I cruise in high gear, but I'm aware that at any time I can shift down to a slower speed. I control the flow of energy at all times.

And when my day is done, I reverse the process and start slowing down. When in the morning I geared up my speed, now I gear myself down to a quiet idle. For now my work is done and I tune down the engine. Now I take time to reflect on the day and be thankful that I did the best I could.

I visualize myself as always in complete control, aware of what I'm doing and why. I see myself taking short relaxation breaks during the activities of the day. I hear friends and fellow workers telling me how calm and yet more efficient I have become. I feel myself taking a few minutes to step back and think before doing a new job so that I need not waste time or steps. Then, I feel myself step forward and carefully use my time and energy in the most efficient ways. I plant in my mind a vivid image or symbol of my success, and I experience this goal-image as already accomplished. I am picturing a positive end result.

After taking daily relaxation breaks, I am far more dynamic and productive when I open my eyes and take action. The more I am asked to do, the more ability I have to do it with and do it in a calm, assured, and positive way.

Thunderstorm Appreciation

Yes, thunder is loud. Its booming seems to go right through you, and flashes of lightning are unexpected. This is something you are already aware of.

Perhaps there was a time long ago in your past, perhaps when you were a very small child, that there was a severe thunderstorm. Being so young and inexperienced, it was natural for you to be unsure of something you couldn't understand. But you knew something was happening.

All of a sudden the world became dark, and loud sounds filled the air. Unexpected light came from nowhere, and the wind rushed through the trees. Children look to the adults in their lives to explain their world to them. Naturally, you looked for assurance from those close to you that everything would be all right.

Perhaps there was no one there to explain this natural phenomenon to you, and to tell you that "Yes, a thunderstorm is powerful and intense, but there is an inherent beauty in it as well. Nature is cleaning the air and putting on a light show, complete with sound effects." It could be that the adult with you at that time had an unreasonable feeling about storms and could not assure you and calm your feelings. Whatever the reason or situation, that was long ago and in the distant past. Here and now with your present understanding you can take another look and feel better about changing your perspectives.

All that is important is that you are willing to change.

Sometimes old feelings actually create more stress than the thing feared. Fear can be good when it allows caution in your life, so you don't take foolish chances. By understanding and restructuring your thought patterns you can create feelings of a healthy respect for nature. It is time to change the pattern. Visualize and feel yourself actually enjoying nature's light show. Let the heavens declare their majesty; it is for your listening and visual pleasure. Focus on a clear picture, create a vivid symbol that brings a new message to your inner mind. Involve new feelings and positive emotion— plant a new seed. It has been said that there has to be rain before there can be a rainbow, so use the rainbow as your emblem of success, your goal-image. (Pause) And feel this feeling of ease as already accomplished.

Pain Alleviation/Hypnoanesthesia

<u>Common Uses & Depths:</u>

1) Glove Anesthesia- minor surgical procedures; light to medium trance
2) Displacement- minor surgery; minor chronic pain; light to medium trance
3) Hypnoanesthetic Key- elderly clients; chronic pain, medium to deep trance
4) Dissociation- many surgeries; medium to deep trance
5) Light & Dimmer Switch- many surgeries; chronic pain; medium to deep trance
6) Shrink A Symbol/Color Healing- headaches & chronic pain; light to medium trance

Glove Anesthesia

...now I want you to remember a time when one of your hands or whole arm went numb. Imagine that clearly and hold your hand out in front of you. Support the weight of your arm by resting your elbow on something... Holding your hand out, and still relaxing easily and deeply, you will imagine the hand being so numb that it will start to tingle. You will feel tingling in your finger tips. You feel tingling in your hand, as if it has an anesthetic glove on it. This is a sign that it is going numb now as you relax, letting the hand fall asleep now, falling asleep, numb. Feel the numbness in the finger tips. You can transfer this numbness easily and effortlessly to any part of your body and when you stroke your _____, the numbness will transfer and it will also go numb. The _____ will receive the numbness and go numb, feeling very little. You will be able to do this in the future by relaxing yourself (listening to a tape or CD or doing self hypnosis) remembering when your hand was numb, transfer the numbness and feel nothing but a little vibration, or simply feel nothing...

(Optional test) You can test that part of the body now by reaching over and pinching the skin with your fingernail and notice how you feel very little sensation, very little or nothing at all. It's numb, you're numb. You're relaxed, relaxed more deeply now.

Displacement

...and now I want you to imagine where your discomfort is. You will imagine the discomfort moving now. It is going to begin to move from your_____ down toward the floor. It moves half way down to the floor and begins to drift through your_____. From there it moves all the way down through the tip of your toes and onto the floor. It's moving into the floor now, heavy, soaking in. It melts into the floor and stays there now. It stays deeply embedded into the floor.

Hypnoanesthetic Key

... and now I want you to continue to go deep, very deep, to your deepest level (pause). You are very deeply relaxed, very deep. Now I want you to pull on your wrist and say the word, "Deep" to yourself (pause). Next, say to yourself, "Relaxed." At that time, you will imagine a favorite activity. For the next couple of minutes, you will imagine a favorite activity very clearly (pause). (May want to question client to make sure they are in a favorite activity). Next I want you to pull on your wrist again and say to yourself, "Wide awake and feeling good." Then you will open your eyes and awaken. (End)
(Suggest that the client listen to these instructions by tape or CD for a while, until they can do it without the tape or CD, starting with a wrist pull and the word, "deep." Monitor results.)

Dissociation

Imagine that the part of the body that was uncomfortable no longer belongs to you. You are cutting off all of the sensation and awareness to your_____ now, and you simply tell yourself that this part of your body doesn't belong to you anymore. It is detached from your body awareness. It is separate from you now, so you feel nothing there anymore... let it disappear.

Light & Dimmer Switch

Imagine that there are wires that run from your_____ to your brain, to your mind. These wires carry all of the nerves, all of the sensation between your_____ and your mind. Imagine that you also have a box somewhere in the middle of these wires with switches in it. You are going to click off each of these switches now. Click off each of these switches one-by-one until virtually all of the sensation to your_____ is disconnected. You feel less, and less vibration from that part of the body. Less, and less, and less, until you are more and more comfortable. Comfortable now. Comfortable.

Shrink A Symbol/Color Healing

Imagine that your discomfort has a shape now. Notice what shape that is. (Ask & get feedback.) Shrink this symbol of your discomfort down until it's the size of a baseball... further down now until it's the size of a golf ball. Now change it to a color that represents healing for you, a healing color. This is one of your favorite colors now as it gets brighter, and brighter. (Ask & get feedback.)
Now shrink it down until it's the size of a marble... further down to the size of a pea... smaller now until it's the size of a small bead... further down until it's the size of a pin head.... now until it's the size of a speck of dust. And then you may notice that you are able to feel a small breeze or gust of wind and you will feel the dust get blown out of the body and onto the floor. It's gone now; you feel fine. You feel fine.

Count Back Regression

"OK, now I want you to imagine which direction your subconscious mind stores the past. Your past memories could be located above you, beside you, in front or behind you. I want you to allow yourself to float back into that direction now, leaving the present behind... I will count from one to five, and I want you to allow yourself to float back over as many years as necessary to find (state the cause of the problem, or the goal). One... leaving the present and floating back toward the direction of the past. Two... floating back over the years. Three... farther back and more deeply relaxed. Four... approaching the (goal)...and you're there now at the number Five."

Time Tunnel Regression

(To be done at the end of the stairs deepening technique.) "At the end of the stairs there's a doorway marked memories. When you open the doorway there is a long tunnel with a light at the end of it symbolizing birth. You begin to walk down the tunnel and there are windows from different scenes of you life. In the windows you notice yourself as being younger and younger. You may go back as far as is necessary for (goal of session). You will either float through a window or float through the bright light at the end of the tunnel and you will be there. When I count from one to five, you will be there. One...two...three...four...five."

Open Ended Regression

"When I count from one to five, you will go back to the cause of the problem. Simply trust whatever your subconscious mind brings you. Whatever it shows you will be the source of the problem. One...two...three...four...five."

Affect Bridge

"Okay, close your eyes and concentrate on that feeling and keep describing it....(client describes further) Now I want you to allow that feeling to float back into the direction of the past where your unconscious mind stores past memories and images. Take this feeling back to the first time you ever felt this way, the source of this feeling, when I count from one to five... One, floating back over the years, Two, farther, Three, back to the source of the problem, Four, (pause)... and Five."

Timeline Regression

"OK, I want you to allow your mind to drift and wander. Allow it to drift up above your body as you surround your body with the white light from the highest source. This light is safe and protective. As the light gets closer it surrounds you and you are able to float up above the room, noticing us down below. Allow the mind to drift up higher and lighter until you go up above the building... and even further up to where the building we are in is very tiny. Now surround the present moment with white light as it stands for change and transformation. Then shrink it down until it's a small white ball. Then draw a white line through the present moment way into the past, and way into the future (pause). And rise up above your time line so that you can see how far it extends out into both directions, way into the past and way into the future from here (pause). Then allow yourself to float into the direction of the past along your time line as I count from one to five. When I reach the number five you will go into the time line and experience the source of the problem... One, floating back, two, farther, three (pause), four, down into the source... at the number five."

Cloud Regression

I want you to now imagine you are in a beautiful place looking up at the clouds. One of the clouds begins to drift down towards you. Soon, you feel it moving over your body, feeling it beginning to lift you up higher and lighter into the beautiful blue sky. You are relaxed and at ease. Soon you are drifting into space, moving out of the earth's atmosphere. You look into the distance and see a beautiful, glowing star. You are drawn to this star and begin to float in to it. I will count from one to five and when I get to five you will be within this star. 1 - moving closer, 2 - relaxed, 3 - a little closer, 4 - almost there, and 5 - you are there. You look in front of you and see a long hallway as the cloud sets you down. In this hallway are 5 doors. As I count from 1 to 5 you will choose one of these doors to open. This door will take you into another time in your life. Take your time and look at each door and choose the one you wish to open. 1-2-3-4-5. You have opened the door. Now I want you to now tell me where you are and what you are seeing.

Age Regression—Complete Session

(Induction:)
(Safe Place Imagery)

"Separate your hands and feet and put your back into a comfortable position that it can stay in for a long period of time. Close your eyes and allow yourself to imagine a safe place in nature where you've been before or plan to be in the future; or you may just create it within yourself. Brighten up the color and notice how clear it is and how good it feels to be there. Notice the things that are moving about and how peaceful and wonderful the mood is. Hear the sounds of nature now, as they get a little louder. You may feel the warmth of the light in the sky, and the coolness of a gentle breeze. There may be a familiar pleasant scent in the air...a few clouds drifting gently across the sky, a sky that goes on forever, and a bright light that reaches you shining down between the clouds...allowing you to feel warm and relaxed. This light stands for everything that's good in life, such as love, peace, serenity, tranquility, and pure relaxation."

(Progressive relaxation)

"Allow this light to flow through you relaxing every muscle fiber, cell and tissue. As it flows through you from head to toe, allow it to completely relax each muscle group. As it begins to flow through the forehead, feel the stress lines simply spread apart. It automatically continues to flow through the eyes as the thread muscles behind the eyes simply unravel and the eyes get heavier. The white light automatically continues to flow down over the temples and through the front of the neck...at the same time down the back of the head, neck and shoulders. Allow gravity to pull the shoulders down into their natural position. The mind may wander and drift, or it may become drowsy and foggy. Whatever happens is completely natural; you'll still hear the relaxing sound of my voice, which is soon to become a comfortable feeling in the background. My words will soon blend into one another and flow into your mind naturally, so you'll be free from having to listen to the words as the subconscious will recognize what they mean anyway. Now the mind simply unwinds like a big spring...letting go. As the sun rises on one side of the earth and sets on the other, each day is similar to one another with common themes. Each day has learning lessons of its own, regardless of the ups and down, moods, stresses...it has nothing to do with this. This is just pure-simple relaxation. All fears, guilts and self blame are released. Problems, pressures, and stresses built up through time are useless and unnecessary.

Allow the white light to continue to flow through the elbows, wrists, and out the fingers. You may notice a tingling sensation within the hands which further shows you're beginning to relax as the bodily functions are slowing down. The breathing becomes a shade deeper; with each more relaxing breath, feel the body rest more firmly against the pads that you're laying or sitting against. As the white light flows down through the back, all the muscles and tendons wrapped around the vertebrae unwind, and the back settles into its natural position automatically. The light flows through the waist, knees, ankles, and out through the toes, pushing out all stress, concerns, worries, in the form of tension or tightness, which may have been locked up in the body and are useless to us now. Feel the nerves dimming, like dimming the lights. With each beat of the heart, you're naturally more in touch from becoming relaxed in this way, allowing yourself to go deeper into relaxation. Feel all the muscles and tendons droop and hang on the bone structure, loose and limp."

(Deepening techniques)

(Numbers Script) "OK now, when I count from one to ten, you will go one thousand times deeper, one hundred times deeper with each number you hear without even trying. One, and one hundred times deeper. Two, two hundred. Three...farther. Four...four hundred. Five...deeper. Six...(pause) Seven....and seven hundred. Eight...deeper. Nine...(pause) and Ten... one thousand times more deeply relaxed."

(Floating Script) "Imagine that you are floating to your deepest level. Because you know where that deepest level is, you will simply feel yourself float there when I count from one to five. One, floating. Two, farther. Three, more relaxed. Four, deeper. And Five, deeply relaxed."

(Count Back Regression)

"OK, now I want you to imagine which direction your subconscious mind stores the past. Your past memories could be located above you, beside you, in front or behind you. I want you to allow yourself to float back into that direction now, leaving the present behind... I will count from one to five, and I want you to allow yourself to float back over as many years as necessary to find (state the cause of the problem, or the goal). One... leaving the present and floating back toward the direction of the past. Two... floating back over the years. Three... farther back and more deeply relaxed. Four... approaching the (goal)...and you're there now at the number Five."

(Open Ended Questions)

"What are you aware of?"   (pause for answer)
"What's happening?"   (pause for answer)
"What happens next?"   (pause for answer)
"And then what happens?"   (pause for answer)
"What else are you aware of?" (pause for answer)

(Optional: for therapy, continue to use the following paragraph several times; for an exploration exercise, skip and go to higher self integration below.)

"Go to the next significant event when I count from one to three..
one...two...three..." (pause for 1/2 to 1 minute)
"What are you aware of?"   (pause for answer)
"What's happening?"   (pause for answer)
"What happens next?"   (pause for answer)
"And then what happens?"   (pause for answer)
"What else are you aware of?" (pause for answer)
(Apply Transformational Model Here (e.g. wounded child blending, integrating past and present content, etc.)

(Optional Higher Self/Spirit Guidance Therapy Model)

"Now I want you to continue floating upward above the memory...floating into the higher light where you will encounter spirit guidance and/or a message from your higher self as to the purpose for having had this memory at this time, when I count from one to three. One...two...three.
(1-2min. pause) Can you relay to me what that message is?"

(Reorientation)

"Okay, now, I want you to simply float above that memory and start letting your mind drift back toward the present moment, leaving the past behind. (pause) Floating back into the present moment and feeling fine." (pause)

(Awakening Procedures)

"And now I'm going to count back from 5 to 1 and when I reach the number 1, you can then come back completely into your body and normalize.
Five...You'll remember everything you have experienced.
Four...Bringing back a beautiful sense of well-being.
Three...More in touch with the room around you.
Two...The mind and the body are returning back toward normal.
When you imagine the number *One*...in your mind's eye within the next
minute, you'll become wide awake, refreshed, and feeling good."

Past-life Regression—Complete Session

(Induction)
(White Light Imagery)

    Separate your hands and feet and put your back into a comfortable position that it can stay in for a long period of time. Close your eyes and allow yourself to imagine a beautiful light emanating from the highest source in the universe...the brightest, highest, most pure light from the most beautiful and peaceful place. You know where this place is and can draw this light to you. You can feel yourself being drawn into the light as well. This light stands for everything that's good in life and beyond, such as unconditional love, peace, serenity, tranquility, and pure relaxation. Experiencing this wonderful light is your birth right, as you are from this place. Now you may safely unite with the vibrations of the light.

(Progressive relaxation)

    Allow this beautiful light to flow through every part of your being. As it flows through you from head to toe, allow it to completely relax every muscle. As it begins to flow through the forehead , feel that area simply relax. It automatically flows through the facial muscles and continues to flow down over the temples and through the front of the neck...at the same time down the back of the head, neck and shoulders. Allow gravity to pull the shoulders down into their natural position. The mind may wander and drift, or it may become drowsy and foggy. Whatever happens is completely natural; you'll still hear the relaxing sound of my voice which is soon to become a comfortable feeling in the background. My words will soon blend into one another and flow into your mind naturally, so you'll be free from having to listen to the words as the subconscious will recognize what they mean anyway. Imagine that the mind is like a big whirlpool full of thoughts that have been swirling around, and now you can pull the plug and let those thoughts just drift and drain away.

    Allow the white light to continue to flow through the arms and out the hands. The breathing becomes a shade deeper. With each more relaxing breath, feel the body resting with a safe deeper, more peaceful sense of relaxation. As the white light flows down through the back, all the muscles and tendons wrapped around the vertebrae unwind and the back settles into its natural position automatically. As it flows through the center of your being, notice that the light within you grows brighter and brighter. The part that has come from the light from within your center is now filling you and then emanating from you, as it intensifies. Feel your light surrounding you now with the light from the highest source. The light continues to flow through the waist, knees, ankles, and out through the toes. You and the light are one now...flowing within the same higher vibration.

(Deepening techniques)

    (Numbers Script) "OK now, when I count from one to ten, you will go one thousand times deeper, one hundred times deeper with each number you hear without even trying. One, and one hundred times deeper. Two, two hundred. Three...farther. Four...four hundred. Five...deeper. Six...(pause) Seven....and seven hundred. Eight...deeper. Nine...(pause) and Ten... one thousand times more deeply relaxed."

(Floating Script) "Imagine that you are floating to your deepest level. Because you know where that deepest level is, you will simply feel yourself float there when I count from one to five. One, floating. two, farther. three, more relaxed. four, deeper. And five, deeply relaxed."

(Time Line Regression)

"OK, I want you to allow your mind to drift and wander. Allow it to drift up above your body as you surround your body with the white light from the highest source. This light is safe and protective. As the light gets closer it surrounds you and you are able to float up above the room, noticing us down below. Allow the mind to drift up higher and lighter until you go up above the building... and even further up to where the building we are in is very tiny. Now surround the present moment with white light, as it stands for change and transformation, then shrink it down until it's a small white ball. Now draw a white line through the present moment way into the past, and way into the future (pause). Now feel yourself float up above your time line so that you can see how far it extends out into both directions...way into the past and way into the future from here (pause). Allow yourself to float into the direction of the past, floating back over that past year and further, over the age of ____(nearest decade then pause)... further back, over the age of 20 (pause) (Option: unless the client has had a successful childhood age regression previously, stop at a positive one here for a brief review)... 15... 10...9...8...7...6...5...4...3...2...1 ...through birth and to the other side. You may experience a flash of light, or a grey or violet area...just keep floating back through that place and when I count from 1 to 5 and reach the number 5, you will be (state therapeutic goal or...) float down into your time line into another place and time...a past life that is most beneficial for you to experience at this time. One...floating back, two...farther, three...way back , four... floating into another place and time on the time line.. and you are there now at the number five."

(Open Ended Questions)

"Look down and tell me what you're wearing." (pause for answer)
"What are you aware of?"   (pause for answer)
"What's happening?"   (pause for answer)
"What happens next?"   (pause for answer)
"And then what happens?" (pause for answer)
"What else are you aware of?" (pause for answer)

"Okay. Now, I want you to go to the most significant event in this lifetime when I count from one to three..one...two...three..." (pause for 1/2 to 1 minute)
"What are you aware of?"   (pause for answer)
"What's happening?"   (pause for answer)
"What happens next?"   (pause for answer)
"And then what happens?" (pause for answer)
"What else are you aware of?" (pause for answer)

(Optional research methods- if memories are clear, ask name, date, or place below)
"What name comes to mind?"
"What time era does it seem like?" (Optional: for research, seek out a newspaper)
"What part of the world does this seem like?" (Optional: for research, seek out a map)

"All right, now, I want you to go to the last day, to the final moments of your life, when I count from one to three...one...two...three..." (pause for 1/2 to 1 minute)

 "What are you aware of?" (pause for answer)

 "What's happening?" (pause for answer)

 "What happens next?" (pause for answer)

 "And then what happens?" (pause for answer)

 "What else are you aware of?" (pause for answer)

 "Before you leave this body, think of the condition it is in...and if there are any physical residues in the current body of the present life." (pause for answer)

 Think of any mental decisions you made that may be still with you in the present life" (pause for answer)

 "Now, as you are leaving this body, think of any emotions you took with you from that lifetime" (pause for answer)

 "What were the lessons learned?" (pause for answer)

(Optional Visual Emotional Clearing Therapy Model)

 "Okay, now allow yourself to release all of these residues that have been carried over into the present by floating up above the memory and imagining that the mental, emotional, and physical residues are like a dark metallic dust in the memory; and with the power of your higher self I want you to take a big strong magnet and pull out all the black dust onto the end of the magnet. (pause) Have you done that? (wait for a 'yes') OK, now I want you to take that big black ball off of the end of the magnet and hurl it into space so that it goes way out into space until it burns up into the sun or a distant star."

(Optional Higher Self/Spirit Guidance Therapy Model)

 "Now I want you to continue floating upward above the memory...floating into the higher light where you will encounter spirit guidance and/or a message from your higher self as to the purpose for having had this memory at this time, when I count from one to three. One..two...three. (1-2min. pause) You may relay to me now...what that message is."

(Reorientation)

 "Okay, now, I want you to simply float away from that place and start letting your mind drift back toward the present moment, leaving the past behind. (pause) Floating back along the line of light into the present moment bringing your memories and insights with you." (pause)

(Awakening Procedures)

 "Now I'm going to count back from 5 to 1 and when I reach the number 1, you can then come back completely into your body and normalize.

 Five...You'll remember everything you have experienced.

 Four...Bringing back all the memories and a beautiful sense of well-being

 Three...More in touch with the room around you.

 Two...The mind and the body are returning back toward normal.

 When you imagine the number *One*...in your mind's eye within the next

 minute, you'll become wide awake, refreshed, relaxed, and feeling good."

Akashic Records to Past Life Regression

Remember, with each breath you are going 100 times deeper and deeper and 100 times more relaxed. Allow yourself to imagine that there is a beautiful light emanating from the highest source in the universe. This light is incredibly beautiful and the most peaceful, relaxing thing you have ever experienced. This light beckons you to join it and unite with its serene, peaceful, tranquil vibrations but you cannot quite yet. As the light gently warms your face, you feel all the tension dissolve from around your eyes, face and jaw. You can feel your whole head relax and the tension drains relaxing you more than you have ever relaxed before. The light warms your neck and you feel all the muscles release. As the light reaches your chest there is an immediate release that continues down your abdomen to your pelvis. Every muscle releases and you know you are going deeper and deeper into relaxation with each breath. Your thighs begin to feel the serene, peaceful, tranquil vibrations as the final bit of tension and stress release from your calves and feet. You are now completely and totally relaxed.

Now as your body continues to be totally relaxed, allow yourself to imagine that your awareness is getting lighter and lighter. Deeply relaxed body... lighter and lighter for your awareness. Now imagine that your awareness becomes so light that it begins to comfortably float just above your body that remains deeply relaxed. You find this feeling of floating completely peaceful as the light's vibrations meld with your awareness. You become aware of the most wonderful feeling of unconditional love that totally surrounds you. Realizing that the light is the source of the unconditional love, it begins to draw you to it. You gently float toward the light and you find that it pulls you through a sort of tunnel until you find that you are inside this beautiful light.

As you become accustomed to this place, you realize that everything here is filled with this loving, beautiful light, and there are the most beautiful colors that you have ever seen. There is a scent in the air from the incredibly beautiful flowers. You know you have smelled it before, but you don't recall how or when. You have found a new world of light and beauty.

In front of you, see a massive building. It appears to be a huge cathedral or temple. Somehow you know it is a place of reverence. There are 10 inviting marble stairs that lead to a landing with rows of massive marble pillars on either side of a huge wooden door. Above the pillars is the roof and you notice that it says "Hall of Knowledge" above the majestic entrance. You are drawn to the inviting door and begin to climb the safe stairs. With each step you become more and more comfortable and peaceful. You know that when you reach the top stair you will be totally peaceful and totally calm. You count the stairs. One...more peaceful and calm two...three...more peace...more calm. Four...five...six... More peaceful now. Seven...eight....More calm now. Nine...ten... You are totally at peace and perfectly calm now.

When you walk across the landing, your hand gently reaches out and touches the smooth surface of the pillar and you feel the cool, slippery texture as you pass by. When you reach the oversized wooden door you touch the large golden doorknob and you instantly know that this place contains all the knowledge ever discovered in the past, present, and future. You barely push the door and it opens invitingly so you step in and look around. You hear the door gently close behind you but the sound reverberates and echoes through the long halls that are open before you. You notice the huge vaulted ceilings supported by massive marble columns lighted by beautifully intricate stained glass windows. Walking to the next hall, you turn left and eventually come to a doorway with a safe, inviting stairway down. Above the doorway is a sign that says "Akashic Records".

Your anticipation is rising because somehow you know that you will finally have complete understanding and that makes you more calm and peaceful. The stairs are well-worn marble and they lead you safely to the bottom. There you meet an older man with white hair and a long black robe that reaches almost to the floor. Your unconscious mind is deciding what it is that you need to learn today. He is expecting you, he welcomes you warmly, and you tell him what you need. He nods in reverence and motions for you to sit at one of the many tables. You look to your right, left, forward and behind you and as far as you can see in all directions are rows and rows of bookshelves filled with leather bound books. He returns shortly with several of the leather bound books, and he sets them on the table in front of you. He leaves you alone. You take one of the books. You notice the name on the cover. As you open it, you feel the soft leather of the cover on your fingers. Looking in, you are surprised to find that instead of pages, there are moving images like on a movie screen. The images are strangely familiar and are pulling you into them. You find yourself actually becoming part of the images, experiencing the feelings, emotions, joys and sorrows. You can see, hear, feel, taste and smell everything that is happening. You know that at any time you wish, you will be able to step back and become only an observer to the scenes. Now watch what is happening...

Blue Mist Past-Life Regression

Designed by Henry Leo Bolduc
Revised by Marjorie Reynolds & Allen Chips

Before we start, make yourself comfortable. Relax and feel at ease.

Now that you are ready, you may look forward or upward. You may look at something specific or you may look anywhere, in general. I am going to count down slowly from one to ten, and with every descending number, just slowly blink your eyes. Just think in slow motion with each number.

One. Do it slowly.
Two. That's good.
Three. (Pause for two seconds)
Four.(")
Five. (")
Six. (")
Seven. (")
Eight. (")
Nine. (")
And Ten.

Now, just close your eyes and I'll explain why we did that exercise. We are doing Progressive Relaxation; we simply relax the different parts of the body sequentially. That exercise was for the purpose of relaxing the eyelids. Right now, in your eyelids, you, perhaps, have a feeling of relaxation or a comfortable, tired feeling. Whatever the feeling you sense, just allow it to multiply, to magnify, and to become greater. It is something that you do; only you can do it for yourself. So, just take your time now. If you feel any slight movements in your eyelids, just remember that it is a natural part of this experience. It is called REM—rapid eye movement— and it is observed in the dream state.

Just allow that feeling of relaxation in your eyelids to move outward, as in imaginary waves or ripples, to the entire facial area. Just feel your face relaxing. Feel the relaxation going outward to the entire head area, relaxing the head. Now, let the relaxation flow down your neck, to your shoulders, down the arms, and into the hands. Sense the relaxation in your hands and fingers.

Take a deep breath, now, and let your lungs fill with relaxation. Allow that relaxation to flow to the stomach, to the spine, slowly down the spine to the hips, to the legs, feet, and all the way to the toes. Feel your entire body filled with relaxation. Now, just slow down a little bit and, mentally, examine your body. Make sure that all parts of your body are relaxed completely.

Now, allow yourself to slow down just a little bit more. With the next count downward from ten to one, just allow yourself to continue to relax. With each descending number, just allow yourself to slow down, to become more still and more centered. At the count of One, you may enter your own natural level of relaxation. Counting rapidly now: ten, nine, eight, seven, six, five, four, three, two, and one.

You are now at your own natural level of relaxation and, from this level, you may move to any other level with complete awareness and you may function at will. You are in complete control at every level of your mind. It is something that you want. It is here and it is now.

Remember, you are in a safe and protected place at this time. If, however, you would like to use the White Light of Protection, a Spirit Guide, a Guardian Angel, or any other special form of protection, then you may do so now. You are in a calm and relaxed place where positive energy is available.

(*Pause a few seconds*)

Now, compare your mind to the surface of a quiet pond. On the surface, everything looks peaceful and still but, below the surface, there is great depth and much is happening. You may think of my voice as a breeze whispering in the trees along the shore.

Take a deep breath, now. Perhaps you notice that a drifting is occurring. Perhaps you feel light or, perhaps, you feel heavy. Your mind is alert although you feel that your body is asleep. You remain completely in control of the process. More and more significance is given to your own inner world, to your own inner experience.

Stored deeply in your unconscious mind are memories of other times and other places. Your conscious mind can reach those memories. By looking deeply in to the recesses of your mind, while in this pleasant state of focused relaxation, you can perceive your inner vision and hear the true voice of your heart. With this attention, comes new understanding, growth, and healing. Later, you may apply this knowledge for self-understanding in your current life. In a moment, now, you will begin a series of exercises that will lead to the recall of memories.

Now, move yourself backward in time, going back, now, to a time when you are about fifteen years old. You are about fifteen years old, now. Choose a memory of that time—any memory you wish to recall.

You will find that it is very easy for you to do so. Choose one specific memory—one specific event—you wish to process from that time.

(*Pause a few seconds*)

Enjoy this event. Perhaps you hear voices. Perhaps you perceive other people near you. The images could be in vivid color as in a cinema movie or they could be black and white or they could be vague outlines. It is possible that you might sense the memory. Just let it happen. Bring the saliva to your mouth and it will help you to speak easily. Let your lips become moist and it will be easy for you to talk about what you are experiencing. Describe what is happening. Just begin when you're ready.

(If no answer, "Now, what do you see or perceive or hear?" Take notes related to the response. Acknowledge a response by saying, "Very good " or any similar response.)

Now, take that memory with you as you continue to move backward to the time when you were about four or five years old. Again, choose a memory and - focus upon it. Reach down deeply and feel it. *(Pause) You* are now four or five years old. *(Pause)* What are you doing? What do you see or hear or sense or perceive? *(If no answer, say, "Just imagine it and let it develop from there.")*

What are you wearing? Who are the people around you? What is going on? *(Continue to take notes. Acknowledge responses and ask, "Is there anything else?)*

Take that memory with you as you continue going back, very quickly, through the years of three, two, and one. Moving back, now, through the time of your birth, go to that safe, warm secure place where you feel surrounded, protected, and loved. *(Pause briefly)*

Now, go beyond that time. Go to a place which appears to be a Blue Mist. *(Pause)* The Blue Mist surrounds you and protects you. The Blue Mist is a time of inner peace, of quiet movement, of gentle sounds, and of easy rhythms. It is a time of renewal and a time of great patience. The Blue Mist is a time without measurement; it is a place without distance, without boundaries. It is a timeless place; a placeless time.

The Blue Mist is, really, the avenue from the heart to the Infinite. Even though you are so very comfortable and happy there, a part of you longs for something more. A part of you longs for activity and experience. That longing grows to become a great desire. The desire guides you to become aware of the horizon or to perceive a long tunnel or to walk down a long corridor. You perceive a light. You realize that the light is good and you begin going, growing toward that light.

You travel toward that light, moving away from the pathway of the intellect and traveling on the pathway of the heart and feelings. Through the avenue of the heart, all things are revealed to you.

Soon, you come into the light. The light warms you, wraps you in protection, and merges with your own inner light—the light of your eternal spirit.

Now, take a deep breath. You are ready to emerge from the light and come to earth. Drifting closer, closer.... Place your feet firmly on the earth in fullness of strength. Your purpose is clear; you know why you are coming to earth.

As you step firmly onto the earth in fullness of strength and in clarity of purpose, note what you are wearing on your feet. Trust the impressions that you receive even though, at first, it might seem like imagination. What do you perceive on your feet?

(If no answer, ask, "What's happening with your feet?" After the answer, say, "Very good" or something similar.)

Going slowly up the body, note what you are wearing. How does it look or feel? See the colors, feel the texture. What do you perceive?

(Pause and record the response.)

Is there anything else?
Do you have anything on your head?
What is the color of your hair?
Do you have anything in your hands?
Are you male or are you female?
What is happening around you?
You are doing very well. Is there anything else?

Now, in your mind's eye, slowly look around you. What do you see, hear, sense, or perceive? Just let the story tell itself.

Describe your home or dwelling place.

Who are the people with you? What are your impressions and feelings about the people? Perhaps there is someone special—someone with whom you have a close bond, an affinity, or a strong connection.
.....very good. Is there anything else?

Now, look for any means of transportation, something that feels familiar when you sit in or on it. What are you or other people using for transportation?

You might like to taste some of the food. Smell the food. Taste it. What are you eating?

Now, listen carefully and you will hear your name being spoken by somebody. What do they call you?

What is your work or profession? What are you learning?

Now, move to the time of an important event in your life—a significant episode.

What is happening? What do you see or feel or sense? What sounds do you hear? Remember to let the story tell itself.

Is there anything else?

Move, now, to another significant time in the life. What is happening now? What are you doing? Is there anything else?

As you pass from that life, float safely and gently above your body and above the life. You are going to that timeless place and placeless time where all things are revealed to you.

From the higher perspective, what were the lessons you learned from that life? How did you gain or grow spiritually? ....What could you have done better? ....What brought you the greatest fulfillment in that life? .... What caused the most sadness or hurt? ....What did you learn or accomplish in that life that can help you in your current life?

In the light of those new discoveries and understandings, please relay a message from your past-life self to your current-life self. What does that past-life self want to say to your current-life self? Just begin speaking when you are ready.

In return, give a message from your current-life self to that past-life self. What does the present day self say to that other part of you? Say the message aloud.

What can you do in your current life that would help to heal and to balance any negative happenings that occurred in that life?

Now, look into the eyes of that past-life self and send your blessings, your love, and your compassion.......Bless that part of you. ......Let it fade. Look into the eyes of everyone you saw, those you loved, and send them your love. And as you are doing this important step—as you bless them and send them your love—release them and let them fade. As they fade, they bless and forgive you. Slowly, let the veil drop—allow the curtain to close. Allow a full healing of that life, of that time. Take the amount of time you need and then indicate when they have faded.

(Pause as needed)

(And) Now, as you prepare for the journey back, you may choose to bring back with you only that which is helpful and beneficial. Bring back something holy or special—a gem of wisdom. Bring back only what you want. You may release other memories, feelings, and impressions and retain in your conscious mind only that which is important, helpful and beneficial for you at this time.

Now, slowly, return through the Blue Mist, traveling on the avenue of the heart, where all things are revealed to you. Bring back the information that you have chosen. Slowly, come back through the years into what we call the current life, the present day and the present location. (*Give day, date, and place*)

As you return, realize that you have done very well. You have opened in trust and in thankfulness. In a little while, when you hear a count system from ten to one, you will reorient yourself fully into the present. After counting back from ten, you will be wide awake, refreshed, and feeling great.

       Counting very slowly,
Ten—step firmly and fully into the present.
Nine—feel total normalization at every level of your being.
Eight—feel the life energies returning to your extremities.
Seven—you may want to move your arms or feet.
Six—remember what you have accomplished.
Five—realize that you have done very well.
Four—You are coming up to your full potential. Eight—reenergizing.
Three—revitalizing, and
Two—slowly, open your eyes.
One—You are wide awake.

       Welcome Back

       (Remember to record and to make notes throughout the session.)

Sexual Fulfillment

If you are a healthy, active being, it is possible for you to discover your total sexual abilities. With new understanding, you can develop a positive mental attitude toward all aspects of an exciting sexual life and a harmonious relationship with your partner. By really understanding and being comfortable with yourself, you do not have to try to fit yourself into somebody else's mold. You can be happy knowing that you are you, at ease and confident with your body.

Trust your feelings and inner judgment as you discover and perfect your approach and style. Sexual growth is a learning and sharing experience and, like love, it grows and develops. It becomes more beautiful and more fulfilling. You can calmly enjoy and appreciate each physical experience as an experience—without trying to analyze or compare, doubt or brag, beg or promise. All you really need to do is slow down and savor the experience as a normal and enjoyable experience.

Instinctively your body knows its own needs and in due time will fulfill them. By using pleasure as your guide, you discover and enjoy once latent desires and abilities. You gain confidence and fulfillment by being creative in your passion. You gain new insight through observation. You can ask yourself questions: "When is passion most enjoyable—day or night?" "Do I prefer dim lights or scented candles, music or silence?" "What is my body saying to me?" "How can I be more understanding?"

People guide each other by learning to grow together—no rules regulate what they choose to share. Lasting satisfaction is not a race to be won or a competition to see who finishes first. For some, the goal is not necessarily orgasm; the real goal is in tender touching, gentle words, and intimate embrace, for fulfillment comes also from the heart. Often the greatest joy is not just in the doing, but by being playful together and truly enjoying each other.

The mutual giving and taking of affection is the secret of sexual harmony. Because there are no time limits, you can take hours for your lighthearted and your serious loving. Perhaps share a glass of good wine and a full body massage while playing your favorite music. Be at ease with yourself and each other. Discuss your needs and wants and, as important, what you enjoy giving and doing. Talk together freely. Touch lightly and touch deeply.

In your creative imagination, envision the kind of relationship that you want. See yourself balanced with equal amounts of give and take, doing and accepting, speaking and listening. Joy and happiness become the symbol and the rhythm of your life.

Clearly visualize you and your partner sharing love, making love. Feel the waves of response. And, most important, see yourselves *after* love-making. Picture this afterglow as the most pleasant part, an emblem of togetherness and peace. Feel yourselves hum with satisfaction and fulfillment.

You are pleased that you both enjoyed each other. In your mind you may hear yourself or your partner saying, "Wow! That was wonderful." And it was. Feel this as already accomplished, and be thankful for the sheer joy of being alive and together.

Men's Creating Joy I

For now, I want you to focus on a swirling motion. Imagine a whirlpool that is swirling around in your mind. In this whirlpool are thoughts of the past that no longer serve you, that keep swirling around, circling, swirling... these thoughts may include religious messages about sex. They may also include unpleasant experiences of the past, guilt, blame, shame, or whatever crosses the mind. Because these are all unnecessary and unnatural messages and experiences that have been standing in your way of your natural God-given right to enjoy yourself, I want you to pull the plug now. Pull the plug and let all of these thoughts from the past just drift and drain away. Let them all get sucked down the drain now as you pull the plug, swirling down and drift and drain away. Every last negative thought just drifts and drains away (pause).

Sex is a simple and natural movement that was meant to be very relaxing for yourself and others but with a unique natural rhythm that naturally moves through your mind and body. It happens naturally without trying. It's a simple concept that will cross your mind as a new interest and the body will respond naturally in its own time. You'll just give it time to do what it wants as you use your imagination more positively. It will respond naturally without even having to think about it. You're going to forget to remember to tell the body to respond and when it's time, it's going to respond naturally; and sometimes it will even happen when you least expect it. It will happen naturally from now on, so you are going to spend more time thinking about the things you enjoy about women (the one you love) and that's all for now. You like women and you may love somebody special, so everything is progressively natural in this way. So now you are going to train your mind to think about many interesting things. Many interesting things. Things about women (your loved one) that interest you when you allow yourself to imagine them. It's simple and enjoyable things that you are going to relax with now. These things will be natural imaginings. These things are easy to imagine now...

Imagine a very relaxing time when you are just enjoying yourself, being with the person (you love) you are naturally attracted to. You like them and there's no pressure for anything... You like them and their body. You like her curves, her smile, her loveliness, her feminineness. Notice what you love about her smell now. Smell her. She smells good. You like the smell of her body. Notice as you are close to her that you like to look at her. You look at her feminine curves. You're free from any responsibility to do anything, but you like to look at certain parts of her body. You are attracted to her body, paying attention to the parts of her body that interest you the most. You like certain things about the way she looks and you are looking at those things and remembering the curves. You like them. You are interested in them.
You like certain things that she says to you. You like to listen to her. You like the sound of her voice. You like to listen to the vibration of her voice. You just like being next to her and listening to her. You savor the sounds of her voice.

You like to taste her body. You like to kiss her and taste her unique taste. You like to be with her and taste her. You like the way she tastes, smells, sounds and looks. You like this person and her body. All five of your senses are awakened around her now. You like this. You imagine touching her more often now. You touch the things you like and it feels natural. You like to touch her in a very loving way, when you feel like you both want to. You touch her in very interesting places and you notice that her body is responding. You like to touch her and her body likes your touch. You like it and you may say things that interest her. You may say nice and interesting things that interest her and your body is beginning to respond naturally. The more time you spend training your senses to her, the more and more your body is responding to hers. You both respond now to this emotional closeness. You are both responding when your bodies tell you to. You wait, but your bodies start responding to each other. You hold off for a while and just experience the five senses, until your bodies respond to each other more. Notice how they start responding more and more often.

110

Men's Creating Joy II

You are going to start out now by clearing your mind. Imagine all of your thoughts and concerns just swirling around in your mind, work, performance, stresses all just swirling around; and you are just going to pull the plug and let those things just drift and drain away... just drift and drain away. Your mind is relaxed more now, more clear... You notice that when you are relaxed you can allow your mind to imagine things and your body has been responding on its own. You have been noticing responses in your body occurring completely on its own. It may be at home, when you are out places, when you are tired or perhaps when you are thinking about (your) woman more often. You are thinking about (your special love) woman more often now and your body is showing you with spontaneous responses that it would like to have sexual intimacy. Sometimes you are thinking about her and sometimes you didn't even know your subconscious mind was thinking about it, but something deeper in your mind triggered something natural in your body. A natural human urge is triggering a natural human body response and you're enjoying it. You like it when your body is telling you that it's time to be intimate. Your body wants you to be intimate at those times and you are relaxed with the whole idea now. You are very, very relaxed with the whole idea. The sex act is a very natural thing, and you're accepting this.

You are about to put your bodily responses and your mind and your positive emotions to use. Your body is responding so naturally, and you continue to remain relaxed mentally, releasing all your cares; you stay cool, calm, relaxing as you get the flush feeling now. You like the flush feeling in your body to where you are beginning to want more of it. The rosy stimulated feeling. Deep down, you really enjoy it, but you're ready for more of it. You want to put your body against hers. You may want to lay with her, right next to her making skin contact, feeling free and natural. You may want to listen to her voice, caress her... feel her... look at her... touch her... smell her... taste her... It's natural to want part of you to become part of her now. Your mind is relaxed with this whole natural idea. This God-given inborn state of arousal is very natural now, (because you love her). You and your body want this and your mind is relaxed with the whole idea. You want to have your body flush against hers and feel a rhythm of love, intimacy, connectedness, pushing yourself into the depths of her soul now and you are flush against her and love every aspect of her now. You love her and you desire to be part of her, to be in her and she naturally wants you to be within her too. She wants you and you want her, and you create a song, dance, a type of rhythm that demonstrates your desire for each other that's very natural, very natural. You both create a rhythm with one another that is unique, flush, hot, rhythmical...breathing more deeply and relaxing with the whole idea. The rhythm gradually becomes more and more intense to where you are one. You are one body and you maintain that rhythm, if you lose it you are determined to find it again. You refuse to lose your rhythm, your oneness. You love this and you keep this rhythm as it builds and builds, and it all naturally happens to a height of emotion. You are reaching a new high. Higher and higher until you....and then she...and you both continue, you both continue to go all the way.

You are speeding everything up at the end; speeding up the thoughts in the mind, and then speeding up the stimulated feeling in the body. You will find the most sensitive position for your body, and key thoughts, words, or a key phrase that will trigger your body, and you are able to release, release, and let go...exercising your right to release yourself into your partner. You speed up your right to let go, let go, and there is a wonderful heightened awareness. There is a wonderful, wonderful mental, physical, emotional and spiritual experience that you have with your partner receiving you. You reach new highs to follow through this time. You are reaching the top of the slope and falling over the top, over the top and down the other side. You are simply floating, simply floating now, as you breathe, you breathe together, holding each other, breathing deeply and you may continue to please your partner in creative ways. Then at the end, you may hold each other laying in each other's arms and feel satisfied. You both are satisfied. You can rest now. You're simply successful at doing what's natural. (Pause)

Men's Lengthening Joy

The first thing that I want you to focus on is a swirling motion. Imagine a whirlpool that is swirling around in your mind. In this whirlpool are thoughts of the past that no longer serve you that keep swirling around, circling, swirling... these thoughts may include religious messages about sex. They may also include unpleasant experiences of the past, guilt, blame, shame, or whatever crosses the mind. Because these are all unnecessary and unnatural messages and experiences that have been standing in your way of your natural God-given right to enjoy yourself, I want you to pull the plug now. Pull the plug and let all of these thoughts from the past just drift and drain away. Let them all get sucked down the drain now as you pull the plug, swirling down and drift and drain away. Every last negative thought just drifts and drains away (pause).

Sex is a simple and natural movement that was meant to be very relaxing for you and another person. Together, you are meant to have a unique natural rhythm that naturally moves through both of you simultaneously within your mind and body. Intimacy happens naturally without trying. If you've been hurried in the past, you are now going to slow yourself down, slowing the mind, and slowing the body will become natural for you from this time forward. If you should ever feel your thoughts rush, you slow them down. You slow them down. You have a right to enter into another person's body with yours. You deserve intimacy, and the one you care about does too.... so you slow your thoughts down even at the start of intimacy. If your thoughts begin to race with concerns, you slow them down by saying to yourself, "Slow down. Relax now. I'm going to slow down and relax everything." And you will breathe deeply, slowly, and rhymically, one breath at a time as you and your partner begin to enjoy your ideas about intimacy. You're relaxed with this whole natural idea now. You could care less about the result, you just want to enjoy yourself with your partner for such a longer, slower, period of time.

Your perception of time will be slower, and you will perceive everything as happening in slow motion. Your partner may even seem to move fast sometimes, but you are going to hold on, slow down, and instruct her to simply slow down, or stop, and enjoy the moment, savor the moment. You can tell your penis to stop, stop and cut off the flow, if you need to, just like you've done during urination in the past when you've had to subtly say to yourself, "stop" or "wait." But then your mind is so slowed down, you notice that it begins to drift to boring things sometimes, but you bring your attention back to your partner's needs, and then sometimes it drifts again. You go numb down there. You will tell your penis now to slow down, relax, until it falls asleep or gets tired.

Imagine that your penis has fallen asleep for now, as your mind drifts off to meaningless things, just like your arm fell asleep one night while you were allowing your mind to drift off during sleep. Let your penis feel that sleepy, relaxed, slowed down numbness. The end of the penis may feel stimulated, but that's a sign that it has also gone numb. It's numb now. And when you are ready to enter your partner, the tip of your penis is still numb, it's sleeping, it's got a tingly numb feeling. Inside your partner you feel the rest of yourself, but the tip is numb. You can tell it to "stop" or "wait" or tell her to "stop" or "wait" and the feeling will pass, then you go numb again. You move, slowly with your right to be in her, but it's numb, and to your own surprise, there is a deadened feeling. Your mind drifts sometimes but you are still responsive to your partner's needs. You move within her for a long, slow, period of time. It's slow, slow, and you feel almost nothing down there, until a long, long, time has passed.

When a long time has passed, you may then feel the need to speed things up. Then, and only then, you will tell your body to bring back the sensitive feeling... become sensitive again, and at the very end, after a long, slow time with your partner, you bring back the sensitive feeling, speeding everything up. Speeding everything up at the end; speeding up the thoughts in the mind, and then speeding up the stimulated feeling in the body. You will find the most sensitive position for your body, and key word, or a key phrase that will trigger your body, and you are able to release, release, and let go... exercising your right to release yourself into your partner. You lengthened your joy and now you can feel confident and relax.

Women's Creating Joy I

The first thing to focus on is a swirling motion. Imagine a whirlpool that is swirling around in your mind. In this whirlpool are thoughts of the past that no longer serve you that keep swirling around, circling, swirling... these thoughts may include religious messages about sex. Unpleasant experiences of the past, guilt, blame, shame, may cross your mind. Because these are all unnecessary, unnatural messages and experiences that have been standing in the way of your natural God-given right to enjoy yourself, I want you to pull the plug now. Pull the plug and let all of these thoughts from the past just drift and drain away. Let them all get pulled down the drain now as you pull the plug, swirling down to drift and drain away. Every last negative thought just drifts and drains away (pause).

Sex is a simple and natural expression that was meant to be very relaxing for yourself and others but with a unique natural rhythm that naturally moves through your mind and body. It happens naturally without trying. It's a simple concept that will cross your mind as a new interest and the body will respond naturally in its own time. You'll just give it time to do what it wants as you use your imagination more positively. It will respond naturally without even having to think about it. You're going to forget to remember to tell your body to respond because it's going to respond naturally, sometimes it will even happen when you least expect it. It will happen naturally from now on, so you are going to spend more time thinking about the things you enjoy about men. You naturally love your partner's physique. So now you are going to train your mind to think about many interesting things about him. Many interesting things. Things about your partner that interest you when you allow yourself to imagine him. It's simple and enjoyable things that you are going to relax with now. These things will be natural imaginings. These things are easy to imagine now...

Imagine a very relaxing time when you are just enjoying yourself, being with the person you love. You like being with him and there's no pressure for anything... You love him and his physique. You like his curves, his smile, and characteristics...Notice what you like about his smell now. Smell him. He smells good. You like the smell of his body. Notice as you are close to him that you like to look at him. You look at his masculine physique. You like to look at certain parts of his body. You are feeling a natural attraction to him as a person, paying attention to the things you like about him that interest you the most. You like certain things about the way he looks and you are looking at those things and remembering them. You like them. You have a natural inborn spiritual interest in him. You deserve to enjoy the sensual things about him.

You like certain things you hear when you are feeling close. You like to listen to aspects of his voice. You like to listen to his breath. You just like being next to him and to listen to things about him. You may also hear a favorite song in your head that adds to the mood.

You like to taste him. His lips and more. You like the way he tastes, smells, sounds and looks. You like getting into the mood and his body. All five of your senses are awakened around him now. You like this. You imagine touching him more often now. You touch the things you like, and it feels good. You like to touch him when you feel like you want to. You touch him in very interesting places and you notice that his body is responding. You like to touch him and his body likes your touch. You like it and you say things that interest him. You say words that heighten your interest and your body is beginning to respond naturally. The more time you spend training your senses, the more and more your body is responding to his. You both respond now emotionally and physically. You are both responding when your bodies tell you to. You wait, but your bodies start responding to each other. You hold off for a while and just play with the senses, until your bodies respond to each other more. They start responding more and more often. You like to think about him and his body. You imagine sexual things more and more often throughout the day and even at night during your dreams. You're simply thinking about it more often and you always put it in a positive light. You think about the things you enjoy more often. You are relaxed with the whole idea.

Women's Creating Joy II

It's time to clear your mind for now. Imagine all of your thoughts and concerns just swirling around in your mind... work, performance stress, past programs from religion or childhood, or whatever... imagine it all just swirling around and you are just going to pull the plug for now and let those things just drift and drain away... just drift and drain away. Your mind is relaxed more now, more clear...

You notice that when you are relaxed you can allow your mind to imagine things and your body has been responding on its own. You have been noticing responses in your body occurring completely on its own when you are feeling emotionally close. It may be at home, when you are out places, when you are tired or perhaps when you are thinking about men more often. You are thinking about your man more often now, and your body is showing you with spontaneous responses that it would like to be intimate with that special somebody. Sometimes you are thinking about him, and sometimes you didn't even know your subconscious mind was thinking about it, but something deeper in your mind triggered something natural in your body. A natural human urge is triggering a natural human response and you like it. You like it when your body is telling you that it's time to be intimate. Your body wants you to be intimate at those times and you are relaxed with the whole idea now...more relaxed with the whole idea. Being sensual is a very natural thing, an innate ability among all women, and you know this on a deeper level, so you're relaxing with the idea now. You realize you deserve this joy...perhaps you've earned it.

You are about to put your naturally occurring bodily responses to use. Your body is responding so naturally, and you continue to remain relaxed, mentally releasing all your cares, you stay cool, calm, and you relax as you get the flush feeling now. You like the flush feeling in your body to where you are beginning to want more of that feeling. The rosy stimulated feeling that it's OK to enjoy. Deep down, you really enjoy it, and you're ready for more of it. It's natural to have an innate desire to put your mind, emotions and physical bodies together. You want to be with him, right next to him, with nothing between you. You want to listen to his voice, caress him...feel him...look at him...touch him...smell him...taste him...You want part of him to become part of you now. Your mind is relaxed with this whole natural idea. This God-given inborn state of arousal that is very natural for you now is preparing your mind and body for natural movements. You and your body want this and your mind is relaxed with the whole idea. You want to have your body flush against his and feel a rhythm of love, intimacy, connectedness, pushing yourself against the depths of his inner being now and you are flush against him and love every aspect of him now. You love him and you crave a deep desire for him to become part of you emotionally and physically, to be flush against him and he simply wants to be with you this natural way too. You create a song, a dance, a type of rhythm that demonstrates your desire for each other that's very natural, very natural. You both create a rhythm with one another that is unique, flush, hot, rhythmical....breathing deeply and relaxing with the whole idea. The rhythm gradually becomes more and more intense to where you are one. You are one body, one blended soul, and you know that this is your spiritual inborn right. You maintain the rhythm. If you start to lose it, you are determined to find it again. You notice key thoughts, words, or phrases that enter your mind and arouse you. You gain your rhythm, your oneness. You love this and you keep this rhythm as it builds, and builds and it all naturally happens to a higher level of emotion. You are reaching a new high. Higher and higher until you....and you both continue. You reach new highs, very, very excited emotionally, mentally and physically. The tension in your body is very natural. You let these tensions be there. You are reaching the top now, and falling over the top, over the top and down the other side like a wonderful ride down a slope. You are exercising your God-given right to release, release yourself physically and emotionally with your partner. You have a right to release all your tensions now, and then you are simply floating, simply floating now, as you breathe, you breathe deeply, holding each other, breathing deeply. Holding each other laying in each other's arms, you feel satisfied because you know that whatever happened was perfect for this time. You both are satisfied with everything for now. You did what's very natural and you can rest..Resting...relaxing...resting. Knowing that you can relax, with more positive and confident messages to yourself.

Attracting A Soul Mate

As you imagine the perfect person for you, you will draw them to you. You will train your mind what to look for during this exercise, and the higher forces will respond to your requests. Your requests will go through your higher power, flow down through the collective unconscious and then into your environment. Your imagination of the perfect soul mate exists, because the perfect person for you exists somewhere... so now I want you to make a list in your mind of all the characteristics that this soul mate has. You can imagine their body type and shape, but just as importantly you will make a list of all of the character traits this person has.

Imagine that you are floating up to a room that has a sign on it with the words, "collective unconscious." You open the door and there are volumes and volumes of information stored in a very large type of library. You notice that there is the request board. Imagine this is a chalk board in the collective unconscious where you can make requests. You pick up a piece of chalk and begin to list all of the character traits you want your soul mate to have. Write word, after word, as I pause for a couple of minutes. (pause)... Now you are leaving the collective unconscious room with your request in writing. You close the door behind you and look back to notice a light in the door. There in the doorway is a person standing in the light as you are walking away from the room and back to the present. The light is bright behind them, you can't see their features too well, because it's so bright, but you begin to feel their presence. You can feel them as you start coming back into the present...

Each time that you listen to this script and do this exercise, your list becomes longer, more specific, and detailed, and you will notice a few physical features, but the light will remain bright behind them, and you will mostly see the light...

Beyond Tomorrow

Be aware of a soft, radiant, white light filtering through your mind. Just become aware now of your consciousness being aware of itself. . .as in a dream within a dream. . .looking into a mirror of time. . . flowing into timeless time.

Feel your entire body floating in a vast, infinite, shoreless sea of glowing white light, an essence so light and luminous that it's like a shining mist. See and feel this gentle, illuminating force. It is your own consciousness and it is linked to universal consciousness.

As you feel this warm energy softly bathing every atom and cell of your being, be aware that you are an eternal spiritual being who uses the mind, emotions, and body as instruments of your will. You have the ability to choose whatever thoughts, emotions, feelings and sensations you direct your awareness to, and in this ability is your free-will as an eternal spiritual being.

Now you are becoming more and more aware of your freedom to go beyond the limits of the physical body. You can progress yourself anywhere in space and time by simply directing your attention there. Time, calendar, and space may be illusions of material limitations in respect to the five senses. Time and calendar are inconsequential in the thoughts and vibratory or outer dimensional forces of your eternal self. As you look within and listen to your inner voice, your intuitive pathways will open to new vision and insight.

You belong to that infinite essence which is beyond time and space, because there is only the eternal *now* as it exists on each level of experience. In the realm of higher consciousness, everything that has ever existed and everything that can ever exist on the physical, emotional or mental levels exists now as a possibility. You have the complete ability to see, hear, and experience all these things and to know them, and to understand them, for what they are. The answers are already deep within you.

With patience you can move through space and time to become aware of events that may be waiting to happen. Allow yourself to go, and feel yourself safely and comfortably going into time—through time— beyond time—above time—to those events which are waiting to be experienced and understood. Your inner mind knows far more than you think it knows. Be intimate with your own mind and, reaching the inner self, venture deep, deep into the gentle recesses of your mind—to a place you have never touched before. This is the storehouse of full knowledge in the still waters of your soul. (Pause)

By opening your mind and trusting your inner impressions, you can move freely through time and space. You may be able to bring back with you insight and understanding that can help you in the present. You can mentally discuss and visually picture what you are doing and what is happening.

Look at what you are wearing in this place. Make a mental note of all that you see. What are you wearing on your feet? What are you hearing? Create vivid symbols and word-images to bring back with you. (Pause)

Now begin the slow and careful journey back through time—into what you call the present. And as you come back through the mist of time, you bring back something that will help you.

Chakra Attunement

Perhaps you are aware that you are becoming deeply centered. In a few minutes you can begin a series of exercises for understanding better your internal energy centers, the endocrine system of your body. You can mentally attune yourself to this ductless gland system, the most protected system in your body. If you take a deep breath and look inward, deep within yourself, you can imagine your consciousness entering into you. Turn inward and mentally look around within yourself. Venture inside your own body. (Pause)

As you begin this awareness exercise, you may sense, feel, see, hear, or have other intuitive abilities. You can perceive your neurohormonal energy centers in the very core of your physical body. The reason they are the most protected is because this is the seat of your real essence, the very center of your being, the source that is the eternal you. Notice that the energy field of each chakra is alive, pulsating and in motion. Now, near the center of your head, visualize or sense a clear bright white light. Picture this light as your pituitary gland; this is your superconsciousness. Its vibration is as Jupiter, a beneficial and expanding influence, a giver of life. Perceive this light as a small light bulb aglow with radiant energy. This is the sacred door to spiritual strength, to idealism, and perfection. (Pause)

Now, back and higher in your head, sense a small gland about the size of the tip of your baby finger. Imagine this as a tiny bulb aglow with a vivid light. Perceive this white light as your pineal gland. This is commonly called the third eye or the eye of wisdom. As you send healing attunement to this area, watch the light become brighter. Its energy vibration is as Mercury; it rules intuition, insight, and your spiritual understanding. (Pause)

As you move to your neck and throat area, you can sense a strong white light emanating there. This is your thyroid, ruled by Uranus, with a vibration of change, genius, and inspiration. As you attune your thyroid and parathyroids, the light grows brighter. This is the receptive light of faith, adaptability and freedom—and a special balancing point of your being. (Pause)

Now, going to the thymus in your mid-chest, sense a vibrant white light that is alive with energy, for this is the center of your nervous system. Here is light for going and growing—it is the builder of order and regeneration. The thymus is commonly called the heart chakra, and you are opening this door to unconditional and non-judgmental love. And because it is influenced by Venus, its vibration is sensitive, beautiful, and loving. Thank your thymus, for it determines the energy supply of your body, and let the light shine brighter. (Pause)

You can continue moving to the upper abdomen, near your stomach, to the solar plexus chakra, the adrenals. You can envision a bright white glow of optimism and inspiration. This is the center of awakening creativity, and, because it is influenced by Mars, it is also the door of your strength. The adrenals are your protection and drive. From here come bursts of high-energy adrenaline. Attune this center and feel its strong vibration. (Pause)

You can now go to your next chakra or energy center located in the lower abdomen. This is called the cells of Leydig. Visualize this area aglow with brilliant white light. Here is the light of wisdom shining with vitality, giving and growing. The cells of Leydig are also called the seat of the soul, for it is here that your sealed memory is stored. Neptune—imaginative and mysterious—watches over this area. The white light becomes as a bright flame, an eternal flame of life, guiding personal expression and positive sensuality. (Pause)

Now you can continue to your reproductive center, the gonads, the generative organs of life. Feel the strong white light of high energy and positive passion. This is the source—the beginning, passion, and action. This center is ruled by Saturn—ego and worldly unions. This is the chakra of new life and the continuity of life. Here is the life force and creative fire. (Pause)

Allow the universal white light to brightly flood into your soul in full vibration. Enjoy this attunement, this oneness, this balance. The more you experience, the more you will understand; and the more you understand, the more will be revealed unto you. And as you ask, so shall it be given. You are given an opportunity for thanksgiving; thank your body, thank your mind, and thank your spirit for this attunement.

Developing Psychic Ability

If you take a deep breath and exhale it very slowly, you can imagine that your breath is like the ocean with the waves coming and going. Perhaps you can hear the music of the waves upon the shore. Watch the waves as you breathe in and breathe out. Imagine that you are lying down, resting upon the shore. You can imagine all the weight leaving your body. Use your imagination, for it is a profound gift to use and enjoy.

Just imagine yourself beginning to float—safely—bit by bit. Allow yourself to float comfortably a little bit above where you are lying. Enjoy yourself rising up and floating in the air.
If you take another breath, you can release pressure and tension that once held you down. And releasing them, you begin to rise a little more—safely and pleasantly.

You may imagine yourself as a sea gull, an eagle, or a dove. Perhaps you are sailing with a hang glider or a helium balloon—the right image will come to you. Rise up on the wings of your mind. Feel yourself soaring, gliding, climbing upward to your higher self. Floating freely in the air, you can observe the world unfolding below you. See the colors of the planet: the blues and greens, the earth tones.

Sense the majesty of the heavens and the panorama of the living universe. Soar and glide to the rhythm of life. Ride the wind and soar higher, higher. You have freed yourself from the earthly bonds that once shackled your mind to convention, self-doubt, and confusion. Feel the quiet radiance of life surrounding you, hear the harmony that is you in tune with creation. Be still, observe, and know.

Glide upward, ever upward, toward understanding, toward light, and toward beauty. Beauty surrounds you in this sanctity of space. Here is where other worlds exist beyond the confines of your everyday mind. And just as a seed contains the promise of fulfillment, so does your mind already contain the promise of greater gifts.

If you choose a path of service to others, you can discover and develop your inner psychic gifts. When you choose to serve others with patience, love, and compassion, you automatically become a channel of blessings. Be aware and alert as the spirit of truth beckons you to new understanding, new directions, and new dimensions. When spirit beckons, follow!— carrying a prayer in your mind and in your heart.

As you let go of old fixed ideas, doubts, and other negative influences, you open the way for new love, patience, and gentleness. The spirit guides you to enjoy the rewards of your new reality. Higher knowledge is usually communicated in silence, so you may choose to go daily into the greater silence within.

Be receptive to the guidance of your universal mind. Your higher mind guides you and protects you, even when you are not consciously aware of it. Grow in the silence of your spiritual self.

Be still and listen. Your higher mind already knows your needs and guides you to live a clear new way each day. Your universal mind guides you to action by giving you gifts of the spirit. I Corinthians says, ". . .the manifestation of the Spirit is given to every man [or woman] to profit withal. For to one is given by the Spirit the word of wisdom; To another the word of knowledge by the same Spirit; To another faith by the same Spirit; to another the gifts of healing. . . to another the working of miracles; to another prophecy; to another discerning of spirits; to another diverse kinds of tongues; to another the interpretation of tongues. But all these worketh that one and the selfsame Spirit, dividing to every [person] severally as he will."
(I Corinthians 12:7-11)

Some people are given more than one psychic gift. You may already have developed several gifts. It is good to apply your gifts and not "to put them under a bushel." Gifts of the spirit can be used often as in Romans 12:6: "Having then gifts differing according to the grace that is given to us, whether prophecy, let us prophesy. "Open wide the door of spirit and rightly use the creative energy that is within you.

One way to determine which are your special intuitive gifts is to try each of them. When you talk with someone, listen—really listen—with your inner ear as well as your outer ears. You may hear things being said at the inner level that are not spoken at the outer levels. Listen also to your inner voice and respond to it.

When you see a person or an event, look—really look— and perceive it with your inner vision. See and understand the workings behind the scenes. Open yourself to all the impressions; look deeper than the surface. If you feel that you may have a gift of healing, use this gift. If you feel that you may have a gift of tongues, use this gift. If you have a gift of prophecy, use this gift to serve others, with their cooperation. Be thankful and use your gifts daily.

Look into the deep recesses of your mind and awaken the silent dreamer. In the inner recesses of your own mind rests all knowledge and ability. The permanent records of life are kept of every act and deed, of all history and all thought, of all medicine and technology, and of all advancements. They are kept in your own consciousness and, as you look deep within, you will see all that exists, that has existed, and will exist. This is already in the recesses of your own mind, your soul-mind. And as you are willing to accept yourself, and as you look deep within, then you see, understand, and perceive this; growing and building toward the light. (Pause)

Now create a picture or vivid symbol of yourself using and applying your gifts of the spirit. Bring your accomplished ideals and goals together into a specific image, and visualize it as already accomplished. (Pause)

Now you can slowly return from your upward flight— returning as a floating feather, circling gently, and landing softly back on the beach. Bringing back something positive and helpful with you. Hear the waves and recall the thoughts, feelings, symbols, and ideas from your journey. You are developing your gifts and learning to use them daily, as you open wide to the new spiritual age that is before you.

(Miscellaneous Script)

Transpersonal Publishing Books

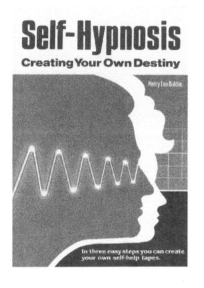

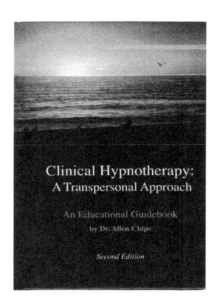

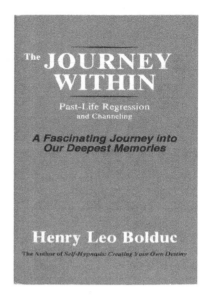

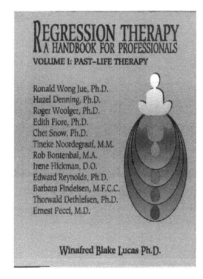

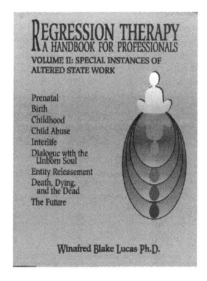

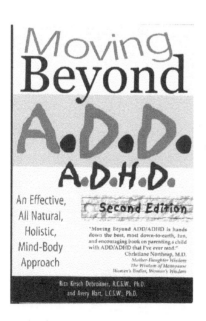

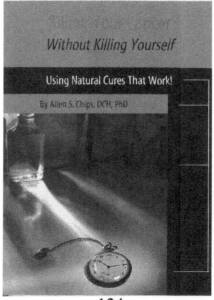

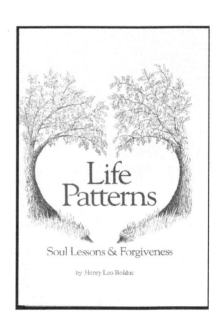

www.TranspersonalPublishing.com

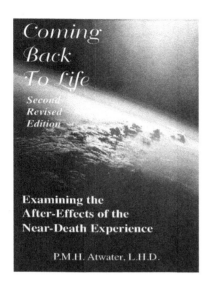

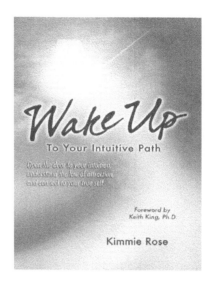

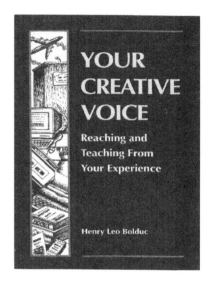

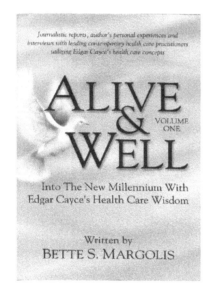

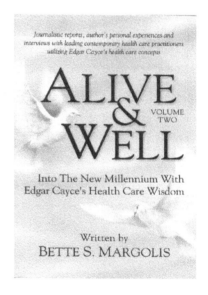

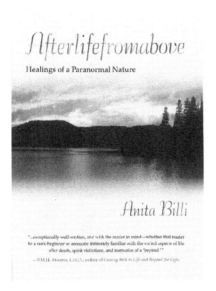

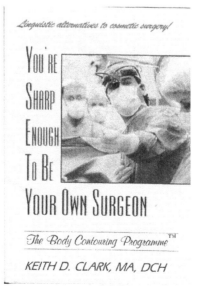

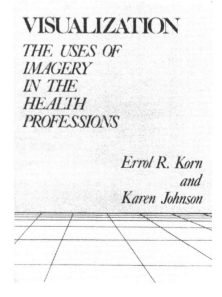

Join Today

The

National Association of Transpersonal Hypnotherapists

Invites You

To Become a Part of The Most Exciting Direction in Hypnotherapy Today

Mail this coupon and your payment to

National Association of
Transpersonal Hypnotherapists
P.O. Box 7220
Kill Devil Hills, NC 27948
800-296-MIND

What Is Transpersonal Hypnotherapy?

Transpersonal hypnotherapy is an orientation that can best be described by defining the word, *transpersonal*- the crossing of mind, body, and spirit or soul. This orientation leads the practitioner into considering a broad scope of interventions that lead to mental, physical or spiritual changes and increased awareness. The transpersonal hypnotherapist allows for client and therapist to address any aspect of the relationship between the mind, body and spirit, and their effects on one another; yet, there is no religious orientation suggested, but instead an unfoldment that makes it possible for clients to explore their relationship to a universal creator and their own unique spiritual walk through human life. One of the primary purposes of NATH and its membership includes educating the public on the higher levels of awareness that hypnosis can bridge one into, in addition to the usual results that are achieved through more traditional clinical hypnotherapy approaches.

Member Benefits and Activities

• Annual Subscription to "The E-Bridge", the quarterly newsletter of NATH, which features articles, benefits, news, and educational development in the field of clinical and transpersonal hypnotherapy.

• Registration Certificate that lets your clients know you are a "Transpersonal Hypnotherapist," practicing with a mind-body-spirit approach.

• Discount on NATH Conferences, several held in the Spring & Fall of each year. These events are worth at least 15 Continuing Education Units (CEUs) each.

• 10% Discount on NATH's Resource Department, a carefully-selected assortment of books and tapes.

• National database registry to include the listing of your practice for incoming NATH referrals.

• Opportunity to form or join regional chapters for networking, camaraderie, and continuing education.

• Liability Insurance for practicing as a "Certified Hypnotherapist." One must be a NATH member to be accepted; refer to the Bridge Newsletter.

126

Membership Requirements & Dues

Certified Members must have earned a Certification in Hypnotherapy from a professional training institution and submit copies of these with the NATH registration coupon or have been practicing hypnotherapy professionally and are willing to submit proof of proficiency in hypnotherapy skills, as per request by the NATH staff. Certified Members use the honor system to obtain 15 professionally related contact hours (CEUs) every year and list these on their renewal form. These may be obtained by reading books, listening to tapes, attending chapter meetings, professional hypnotherapy workshops, and/or hypnotherapy organization's conferences.

Non-Certified Members receive the same benefits as the above except: they do not receive a registration certificate; they aren't listed on the referral directory; and they are not required to submit annual CEUs. Non certified members may upgrade to certified member status once they are certified at no additional charge.

Annual Dues (for either member class)............$70

Registration & Renewal:

Any professional hypnotherapist may register and pay the first year's dues. Approximately 12 months later, members will have the opportunity to rejoin through the mail. Registration certificates are printed around the 15th day of each month.

Two Year Discount:

You may pay the member dues for one year *and* pay next year's dues now and receive a discount on the second year (see registration coupon).

NATH Is A Member of the Council of Professional Hypnosis Organizations (COPHO)

Founded in 1990, COPHO is a cooperative organization of national and international professional hypnosis organizations who seek to maintain high standards in the hypnotherapy profession, provide leadership in the field, and promote inter-organizational unity.

About The NATH Leadership

Allen S. Chips, DCH, *NATH President*
Allen has earned a doctorate in clinical hypnotherapy and a doctorate in the philosophy of natural health. Managing editor for the Bridge Newsletter, official publication for the National Association of Transpersonal Hypnotherapists, and a popular presenter for the Association for Research and Enlightenment on the work of Edgar Cayce. A renowned international instructor of suggestive and regressive hypnotherapy, and author of two textbooks: *Clinical Hypnotherapy: A Transpersonal Approach, Second Edition*, and *Script Magic: A Hypnotherapist's Desk Reference, Second Revised (Lay-Flat) Edition*. Dr. Chips recently released the award-winning book, *Killing Your Cancer Without Killing Yourself: Using Natural Cures That Work!* He serves as President of American Holistic University, an online degree granting institution in holistic arts, hypnotherapy, transpersonal psychology, natural health, and naturopathy.

Dee Chips, B.S.W., M.Ht., C.R.M., *Executive Director*, Cofounder of the National Association of Transpersonal Hypnotherapists (NATH), an experienced Social Worker, a Certified Reiki Master & Trainer, Certified Huna I, NLP and Timeline Therapy Practitioner, and a Certified Master Hypnotherapist. Author of the book, *Inspirational Poetry*. She manages member benefits for the NATH and teaches all of the subtle energy programs (Reiki, Huna, etc...) for the NATH home office.

Honorary Advisory Board

Masud Ansari, PhD, DCH
Ashok Kumar Jain, PhD
Roy Hunter, PhD
Joe Craig, PhD

Philip Holder, PhD
Lawrence Galante, PhD
Henry Leo Bolduc, CHt
Wil Horton, PhD

NATH, PO Box 7220
Kill Devil Hills, NC 27948
800-296-MIND
Web Page: www.holistictree.com
Email: DeeChips@holistictree.com

Yes! I want to join the NATH. Sign me up today...

Name _____ Email _____
(as you want it to appear on your certificate)   (required for newsletter)

Address _____

City _____ State _____ Zip _____

Ofc. Phone _____ Email _____ (for newsletter)

School, Date & Hours of Training _____

Check ____ Money Order ____ Visa ____ MC ____ AmEx ____

Card Number __ __ __ __ __ __ __ __ __ __ __ __ __ __ __ __ Expires ____ / ____

Membership Dues:

Please indicate one or two years...

Certified & Non-Certified Member:
Joining for one year = ($70)................ _____

Two Year Discount Membership:
(To be paid up for a full 2nd year)
......................................*add* $60).............. _____

International Members add $10.................. _____
(& pay by credit card or U.S. money order)

Total $_____

____All new "certified members" must check here and enclose copies of hypnotherapy training certificate(s), or proof of training, with the appropriate fee and this form.

"You cannot teach a man anything; you can only help him find it within himself."
Galileo